**MCRP 6-11C**
**NTTP 1-15M**

# Combat and Operational Stress Control

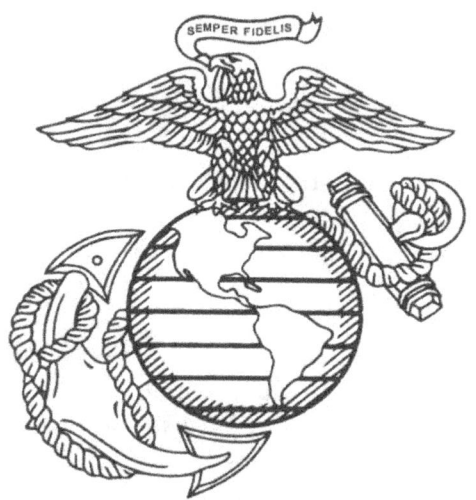

**US Marine Corps**

PCN 144 000083 00
NSN 0411LP1107163

DEPARTMENT OF THE NAVY
Headquarters United States Marine Corps
Washington, D.C. 20380-1775

20 December 2010

FOREWORD

During times of conflict, Navy and Marine Corps leaders are constantly reminded of their duty to lead with military proficiency and to take care of their Marines and Sailors. Ensuring the well-being of Marines and Sailors includes not only strengthening them, but also keeping them strong, monitoring their condition, applying first aid when they are injured, and returning them to full fitness as soon as possible. However, there is much more to caring for our Marines and Sailors than their physical health. Caring for their psychological health is just as crucial. Preserving the psychological health of Service members and their families is as much a warfighting issue as it is a sacred duty and it is of paramount concern to mission readiness.

Leaders in both the Navy and the Marine Corps should use this reference as a tool for teaching and for professional discussion about combat and operational stress control. While we hone technical and physical skills to make us successful in combat and other operations, we cannot neglect the mind and spirit. Marine Corps Reference Publication (MCRP) 6-11C and Navy Tactics, Techniques, and Procedures (NTTP) 1-15M, *Combat and Operational Stress Control*, is not intended to be clinical in nature; rather, it focuses on the leadership responsibilities involved with preserving psychological health in Service members. It provides a foundation so leaders can understand the value of recognizing and addressing combat and operational stress issues and why this skill is so important to the well-being of Marines and Sailors. The effects of appropriate stress treatment reach not only before, during, and after combat and other operations, but also throughout the careers of Marines and Sailors and after their separation from the military. Read this publication. Apply it in your command. It is an important tool to help us strive for a stronger force in the short run and a healthier society in the future.

This publication supersedes MCRP 6-11C and NTTP 1-15M, *Combat Stress*, dated 23 Jun 2000.

BY DIRECTION OF THE CHIEF OF NAVAL OPERATIONS:

WENDI B. CARPENTER
Rear Admiral, U.S. Navy
Commander, Navy Warfare Development Command

BY DIRECTION OF THE COMMANDANT OF THE MARINE CORPS:

GEORGE J. FLYNN
Lieutenant General, U.S. Marine Corps
Deputy Commandant for Combat Development and Integration

Marine Corps Publication Control Number: 144 000083 00

Navy Stock Number: 0411LP1107163

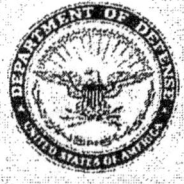

**DEPARTMENT OF THE NAVY**
OFFICE OF THE CHIEF OF NAVAL OPERATIONS
2000 NAVY PENTAGON
WASHINGTON DC 20350-2000

IN REPLY REFER TO:

3510
5 Nov 10

## LETTER OF APPROVAL

1.  NTTP 1-15M/MCRP 6-11C, Combat and Operational Stress Control (COSC) is UNCLASSIFIED.  Handle in accordance with the administrative procedures contained in NTTP 1-01.

2.  NTTP 1-15M/MCRP 6-11C, COSC, is effective upon receipt and supersedes NTTP 1-15/MCRP 6-11C, Combat Stress, dated 23 June 2000.  Destroy superseded material without report.

3.  NTTP 1-15M/MCRP 6-11C, COSC, provides leaders of all grades in both the Navy and Marine Corps a tool for teaching and professional discussion about combat and operational stress control during predeployment preparations, during combat operations, and after combat operations.

4.  NTTP 1-15M/MCRP 6-11C, COSC, is approved for public release; distribution is unlimited.

Approved

*A. M. Robinson, Jr.*

A. M. ROBINSON, JR.
Surgeon General of the Navy (N093)

# TABLE OF CONTENTS

## Chapter 4. Identify: Third Core Function for Leaders

## Chapter 5. Treat: Fourth Core Function for Leaders

## Chapter 6. Reintegrate: Fifth Core Function for Leaders

## Appendices

## Glossary

## References and Related Publications

# 1

# INTRODUCTION TO COMBAT AND OPERATIONAL STRESS CONTROL AND OPERATIONAL STRESS CONTROL

Leaders at all levels are responsible for preserving the psychological health of their Marines, Sailors, and family members, just as they are responsible for preserving their physical health. This responsibility applies to every link in every chain of command from fire team leaders and work center supervisors to combatant commanders and commanding officers. Medical, religious ministry, and other support personnel can help with this task, but only line leaders can balance combat and operational requirements that expose warriors to risks with the imperative to preserve health and readiness.

> *We must ensure the care of our most valuable assets—our Marines and Sailors.*
>
> **Tri-MEF Working Group**

To promote psychological health in their Marines and Sailors, leaders must actively foster resilience, prevent stress problems as much as possible, recognize when stress problems have occurred, and eliminate the stigma associated with getting needed help. Decisions about whether to deploy Marines or Sailors experiencing stress problems or retain them in a deployed status can only be made by operational commanders; however, line leaders can mentor Service members experiencing stress problems toward successful recovery and reintegration.

Psychological health encompasses wellness in body, mind, and spirit. Psychological health is a broad concept that goes far beyond the more limited concepts of mental health and readiness.

Among its many components are a healthy lifestyle, strength of body and mind, moral and spiritual fitness, positive relationships within oneself and others, and confidence based on real competence. Those leadership responsibilities and tasks that directly contribute to psychological health comprise the mission of combat and operational stress control (COSC) in the Marine Corps and operational stress control (OSC) in the Navy. Table 1-1 defines key terms of COSC and OSC.

As an element of force health protection, COSC and OSC have three main goals—prevention, identification, and treatment of stress problems arising from military training and operations. More broadly and simply, the goal of COSC and OSC is resilience, the ability to withstand adversity without becoming significantly affected, as well as the ability to recover quickly and fully from whatever stress-induced distress or impairment has occurred.

| Goals of<br>COSC and OSC |
| --- |
| Prevention<br>Identification<br>Treatment |

| Objectives of<br>COSC and OSC |
| --- |
| Force preservation<br>and readiness |
| Long-term health<br>and well-being |

The two overarching objectives of COSC and OSC are to create and preserve a ready force and to promote the long-term health and well-being of individual Marines and Sailors and their family members. These two objectives are interrelated and are recognized as of paramount strategic importance, since the mission of the Navy and Marine Corps is to win wars and to return good citizens to civilian life after those wars are fought. Taking care of Marines, Sailors, and their families and leaving no one behind are also mandated by the Services' core organizational values.

# The Navy-Marine Corps Combat and Operational Stress Continuum Model

Military commanders and their health and religious ministry advisors have historically taken a somewhat different approach to psychological health protection in operational settings than they have to physical health protection. Whereas timely screening and treatment for injuries and illnesses have always been cornerstones of physical health protection, these same activities have historically been shunned for stress-related problems occurring in operational settings for fear of drawing attention to them and fostering epidemics of stress casualties.

This approach to psychological health protection arose during World War I, when a major conceptual shift regarding combat stress occurred. Prior to 1916, stress casualties, such as "shell shock," were believed to be true medical injuries caused by physical disruption in the brain as a result of nearby artillery blasts. They were treated like any other physical injury, without the burdens of social stigma or personal blame, and many were evacuated from theater on both sides of the war.

Table 1-1. Key Terms of Combat and Operational Stress and Operational Stress Control.

| Term | Definition |
|---|---|
| Combat and operational stress control | Leader actions and responsibilities to promote resilience and psychological health in military units and individuals, including families, exposed to the stress of combat or other military operations. |
| Combat stress | Changes in physical or mental functioning or behavior resulting from the experience of lethal force or its aftermath. These changes can be positive and adaptive or they can be negative, including distress or loss of normal functioning. |
| Mental health | The absence of significant distress or impairment due to mental illness. Mental health is a prerequisite for psychological health. |
| Operational (or occupational) stress control | Leader actions and responsibilities to promote resilience and psychological health in military units and individuals, including family members, exposed to the stress of routine or wartime military operations in noncombat environments. |
| Operational stress | Changes in physical or mental functioning or behavior resulting from the experience or consequences of military operations other than combat, during peacetime or war, and on land, at sea, or in the air. |
| Psychological health | Wellness in mind, body, and spirit. |
| Resilience | The process of preparing for, recovering from, and adjusting to life in the face of stress, adversity, trauma, or tragedy. |
| Stress illness | A diagnosable mental disorder resulting from an unhealed stress injury that worsens over time to cause significant disability in one or more spheres of life. |
| Stress injury | More severe and persistent distress or loss of functioning caused by disruptions to the integrity of the brain, mind, or spirit after exposure to overwhelming stressors. Stress injuries are invisible, but literal, wounds caused by stress, but, like more visible physical wounds, they usually heal, especially if given proper care. |
| Stressor | Any mental or physical challenge or set of challenges. |
| Stress reaction | The common, temporary, and often necessary experience of mild distress or changes in functioning due to stress from any cause. |

After 1916, the medical model of combat stress was replaced by the idea of shell shock. Shell shock was considered a temporary and reversible response to stress that would always resolve with no more than a little rest and encouragement. It was then believed to be caused not by literal damage to the brain, but by a weakness of character brought out by the dangers and hardships of war (see chap. 5 for further discussion). Principles of forward management of stress casualties, based on this new character weakness model, dictated that Service members suffering from stress reactions not be allowed to see themselves as sick, ill, or injured and that they be kept separate from "true" combat casualties. Brief rest and the unwavering expectation that everyone disabled by stress would soon recover and return to the fight—also known as the principle of expectancy—were considered the only tools leaders needed to manage stress casualties.

Medical evaluation and treatment were considered last resorts to be employed only when rest and encouragement failed to get a Service member back into the fight. This historical approach to stress casualties is summarized in *Psychiatric Lessons of War*: "You are neither sick nor a coward. You are just tired and will recover when rested." However, according to *War of Nerves: Soldiers and Psychiatrists*, some of those who failed to recover when rested were executed for cowardice.

The model of combat stress adopted after 1916 succeeded in reducing the rates of medical evacuations from theater for psychological reasons, which is one of the principal reasons this model remained the basis for combat stress control efforts for the rest of the 20th century. Now, seen through the lens of 21st century science, this model had serious shortcomings.

First, it considered only occupational functioning in its definition of psychological health, without sufficient regard for the extent to which less apparent distress or alterations in function may significantly impact current readiness or future health and well-being. During the Vietnam War, for example, stress casualties requiring medical treatment or evacuation were very rare, so combat stress was not then perceived to be a significant force health protection problem. Yet, combat stress must surely have contributed to the in-theater substance abuse, misconduct, and psychological disability after returning to civilian life that have come to characterize that war and its veterans. A significant number of Service members deployed to Operation Iraqi Freedom or Operation Enduring Freedom and exposed to combat or other operational stressors experience persistent, life-altering stress problems during and after deployment, even though most were not recognized as stress casualties in theater. Some postdeployment stress problems may be delayed in onset, surfacing many months after returning from a war zone.

The second problem with the 20th century view of combat stress is that it placed too much responsibility for recognizing and reporting stress problems on individual Marines and Sailors, who may be either unaware of or unwilling to admit to their own psychological problems. The belief that stress problems arising during deployment are not "real" illnesses or injuries and merely "in the minds" of those afflicted has given rise to two comforting, though dangerous, assumptions—that any Service member who is not complaining doesn't need attention and deployed Marines or Sailors who say they are "good to go" after developing stress problems can be safely considered psychologically well and fit without further medical monitoring or care.

The third shortcoming of the 20th century model of combat stress is the degree to which it has intentionally *increased* the social stigma attached to psychological problems of all kinds. The prevailing view, born in part from this character weakness model, has been that only morally weak or unmotivated individuals develop significant problems because of stress. Under this character weakness model, Marines or Sailors who fail to return to full functioning after experiencing combat or operational stress should be considered for an administrative separation for a personality disorder rather than a medical evaluation board. Modern science strongly refutes this view.

While it is true that pre-existing risk factors that contribute to vulnerability for stress-related problems have been identified, everyone is at risk and no one is immune. Studies of the causes of combat-related posttraumatic stress disorder (PTSD), for example, have shown again and again that the degree and frequency of exposure to combat and other intense stressors are a much more powerful determinant of outcome than maturity level, early life experience, or personality style.

Risk factors also exist for physical injuries and illnesses; however, no one would blame individual Marines or Sailors for being injured in a firefight simply because they were not as physically quick or agile as others who escaped injury. Individuals are no more to blame for—or free from the responsibility to acknowledge and cope with—their own stress problems than their own physical injuries and illnesses.

The social stigma surrounding stress problems may have contributed to lower numbers of stressed Service members seeking treatment that might result in medical evacuation, but this stigmatizing conception of combat stress and psychological health has also discouraged Marines and Sailors from ever seeking professional help for stress problems of any kind. Without early treatment, problems are more likely to become chronic and entrenched.

## Combat and Operational Stress Injuries: A Bridging Concept

To address the shortcomings of the 1916 character weakness model, a new concept of combat and operational stress (COS) was developed in the Marine Corps and Navy as being, in some cases, literal wounds to the mind, body, and spirit. These psychological wounds, hereafter called stress injuries, are stages of distress or impairment that are intermediate in severity and persistence. These stages range between stress reactions, which are normal, common, and expected responses to adversity, and stress illnesses, which are less common, but need more medical, spiritual, or mental health treatment to prevent long-term disability.

Just like physical injuries, stress injuries are important indicators of risk—both for being unable to perform normally in some situations and for developing a mental disorder, such as PTSD, if these injuries don't heal completely. There are other parallels between stress injuries and physical injuries—both normally heal over time, both heal faster and more completely with appropriate acknowledgement and care, and neither are the sole fault of the individual. Although physical and stress injuries normally heal, both can leave their mark, signifying lasting change in the area of the injury. Sometimes the scars caused by physical or stress injuries become places of enhanced strength, but sometimes the opposite occurs.

The major differences between physical injuries and stress injuries of great importance to Navy and Marine Corps leaders are that stress injuries are not physically visible, are harder to recognize, and burden their bearer with greater social stigma. They are, therefore, less likely to be voluntarily reported by injured individuals.

The strengths of the stress injury idea as a bridging concept between normal reactions and pathological illnesses are that it—

- Is consistent with 21$^{st}$ century scientific evidence regarding the effects on the brain, body, and mind that is suffering severe or prolonged stress.
- Reduces the burden of stigma associated with persistent stress problems of all kinds.
- Gives leaders a marker of psychological health risk and possible need for early intervention to restore health and wellness.

## A New Approach to Combat and Operational Stress Control and Operational Stress Control

In 2007, the commanding generals of the three Marine expeditionary forces (MEFs) convened a working group of Marine leaders, chaplains, and medical and mental health professionals to develop a new COS model, hereafter called the stress continuum model, for the Marine Corps. Speaking with one voice, the three MEF commanding generals called for a new stress continuum model that would be—

- Unit leader oriented.
- Multidisciplinary.
- Integrated throughout the organization.
- Without stigma.
- Consistent with the warrior ethos.
- Focused on wellness, prevention, and resilience.

The product of this tri-MEF working group was the stress continuum model, outlined in table 1-2 on page 1-8. This model has since become the foundation for all COSC and OSC doctrine, training, surveillance, and interventions in both the Marine Corps and Navy. The stress continuum model is a paradigm that recognizes the entire spectrum of stress responses and outcomes and includes, from left to right, adaptive coping and wellness (color coded Green as the "Ready" Zone), mild and reversible distress or loss of function (the Yellow "Reacting" Zone), more severe and persistent distress or loss of function (the Orange "Injured" Zone), and mental disorders arising from stress and unhealed stress injuries (the Red "Ill" Zone).

reactions and Orange Zone injuries. The further to the right in the stress continuum model individuals are pushed by combat or operational stress—the deeper into the Orange or Red Zones they get—the more medical and mental health professionals become important for returning those individuals to Green Zone wellness. For Marines or Sailors suffering from diagnosable Red Zone mental disorders, such as PTSD, depression, or anxiety, unit leaders remain crucial for recovery and reintegration.

## Green "Ready" Zone

Service members functioning in the Green "Ready" Zone exemplify adaptive coping, optimal functioning, and personal well-being. The Green Zone is not the absence of stress, since the lives of Marines, Sailors, and their family members are seldom without stress. Rather, it is an effective mastery of stress without significant distress or impairment in social or occupational functioning. One important goal of all selection and screening, training, and leadership in the military is to ensure Green Zone readiness or to restore individuals and units to the Green Zone once they have experienced distress or loss of function because of combat or operational stress. The following are some of the attributes and behaviors characteristic of the Green "Ready" Zone:

- Remaining calm and steady.
- Being confident in oneself and others.
- Getting the job done.
- Remaining in control physically, mentally, and emotionally.
- Behaving ethically and morally.
- Sleeping enough.
- Eating well and the right amount.
- Working out and staying fit.
- Retaining a sense of humor.
- Playing well and often.
- Remaining active socially and spiritually.
- Being at peace with oneself.

## Yellow "Reacting" Zone

Service members in the Yellow "Reacting" Zone feel mild and temporary distress or loss of function due to stress. Yellow Zone reactions are always temporary and reversible, although it is hard to know whether they will be temporary and leave no lasting changes while they are occurring. Yellow Zone reactions are common and can be recognized by their duration and relative mildness. Although no research has yet been done on the prevalence of mild and transient distress or loss of function in operational settings, it is likely that such Yellow Zone stress reactions are common for everyone, especially in response to new challenges. From the point of view of stress, all training is designed to enhance skills and abilities through repeated exposure to intentional Yellow Zone situations. Yellow Zone stress reactions are common not only during deployments, but also during predeployment training and preparation and postdeployment homecoming and resetting. The following experiences and behaviors characterize the Yellow "Reacting" Zone:

- Feeling anxious or fearful.
- Feeling sad or angry.
- Worrying.
- Cutting corners on the job.
- Being short tempered or mean.
- Being irritable or grouchy.
- Having trouble falling asleep.
- Eating too much or too little.
- Losing some interest, energy, or enthusiasm.
- Not enjoying usual activities.
- Keeping to oneself.
- Being overly loud or hyperactive.
- Being negative or pessimistic.
- Having diminished capacity for mental focus.

Two defining characteristics of Yellow Zone distress or changes in function are that they are usually mild and always resolve completely as soon as either the challenge that provoked them ends or the individual adapts to the challenge and becomes more accustomed to it. Because Yellow Zone reactions are mild and self-limiting, they don't require professional treatment. Nevertheless, Yellow Zone reactions are important to unit leaders because Marines, Sailors, and family members who are affected by stress in any way are not functioning at their best and are at risk for becoming injured by stress—lapsing into the Orange Zone—if their stress is not mitigated.

## Orange "Injured" Zone

The Orange "Injured" Zone can be defined as encompassing more severe and persistent forms of distress or loss of function that signal the presence of some kind of damage to the mind, brain, or spirit. Whereas Yellow Zone reactions are like a tree branch bending with the wind—always capable of springing back into place once the wind calms—to some extent, Orange Zone injuries are like a branch breaking because it was bent beyond its limits. Like physical injuries, stress injuries occur across a broad spectrum of severity—from mild stress "bruises" that are barely noticeable, to more severe stress "fractures" that may be briefly incapacitating and may not heal without professional treatment. Although stress injuries cannot be completely undone—one can never become "uninjured"—their usual course is to heal over time like physical injuries.

Stress injuries may be recognized in their early stages by the severity of the symptoms they provoke and the intensity of the stressors that cause them. The more lasting nature of stress injuries in the Orange Zone may become apparent over time. Since stress injuries are not mental disorders, clinical mental health expertise is not required to recognize them. Nonetheless, operational commanders and small unit leaders may rely heavily on their chaplains and organic medical and mental health personnel to help identify and treat Orange Zone stress injuries.

Combat operational stress injuries have four different possible mechanisms or causes—

- **Life-threat**. Due to exposure to lethal force or its aftermath in ways that exceed the individual's capacity to cope normally at that moment, life-threatening situations provoke feelings of terror, horror, or helplessness.
- **Loss**. Loss can be felt due to the death of close comrades, leaders, or other cared-for individuals or the loss of relationships, aspects of oneself, or one's possessions by any means.
- **Inner Conflict**. Stress arises due to moral damage from carrying out or bearing witness to acts or failures to act that violate deeply held belief systems.
- **Wear and Tear**. This stress comes from the accumulated effects of smaller stressors over time, such as those from nonoperational sources or lack of sleep, rest, and restoration.

Although stress injuries may be caused by one or more of these four mechanisms, since they often overlap and occur at the same time, the experiences, behaviors, and symptoms that characterize them are similar regardless of mechanism. Symptoms suggesting stress injury include the following:

- Losing control of one's body, emotions, or thinking.
- Having difficulty falling asleep or staying asleep.
- Waking up from recurrent, vivid nightmares.
- Feeling persistent, intense guilt or shame.
- Feeling unusually remorseless or emotionally cold.
- Experiencing attacks of panic or blind rage.
- Losing the ability to remember or think rationally and clearly.
- Being unable to enjoy usually pleasurable activities.
- Losing confidence in previously held moral values.
- Displaying a significant and persistent change in behavior or appearance.
- Harboring serious suicidal or homicidal thoughts.

> The most important distinction for leaders to make is between Yellow Zone stress reactions and Orange Zone stress injuries because those who are injured may not perform as expected and they are at risk for future illnesses.

This distinction between Yellow "Reacting" Zone and Orange "Injured" Zone is the most important judgment that leaders make regarding the stress continuum model for two important reasons: first, Marines, Sailors, or family members who have suffered a stress injury may be significantly impaired in their occupational and social functioning, so they may be no longer fully able to perform their duties as expected or to participate in cohesive military and family units; second, because Orange Zone injuries may not resolve on their own, signs or symptoms of a stress injury should always be considered an indication of the need for further evaluation and possible treatment. All stress injuries deserve to be monitored over time to ensure healing and resolution. The earlier a stress injury receives needed professional attention, the more likely it is to heal quickly and completely.

## Red "Ill" Zone

The Red "Ill" Zone is the zone of diagnosable mental disorders arising in individuals exposed to combat or other operational stressors. Since Red Zone illnesses are clinical mental disorders, they can only be diagnosed by health professionals. Nevertheless, commanders, unit leaders, peers, and family members can and should be aware of the characteristic symptoms of stress illnesses so they can identify them and make appropriate referrals as soon as possible. The most widely recognized stress illness is PTSD (see app. A, *Posttraumatic Stress Disorder Overview*), but stress illnesses may take many different forms, often occurring in the same individual at the same time or at different times. Some other common Red Zone illnesses include the following:

- Depressive disorders, especially major depression.
- Anxiety disorders, including generalized anxiety and panic disorder.
- Substance abuse or dependence.

Specific indicators of the presence of a stress illness—and the need for prompt mental health evaluation—include the following:

- Stress injury symptoms, such as long-lasting and disabling distress or impairment of normal functioning.
- Stress injury symptoms and impairment that do not significantly improve within several weeks of returning from operational deployment.
- Stress injury symptoms and impairment that worsen over time rather than improving.
- Stress injury symptoms and impairment that return after improving or seeming to resolve.

Marines, Sailors, and their leaders may be very reluctant to think that they or someone in their unit may be suffering from a Red Zone stress illness. Many young warriors would rather be told they have cancer than PTSD. Individuals in the Red Zone may deny to themselves that there is a problem at all or they may justify their feelings and behaviors to themselves and family members. They may delay seeking medical care with hope that, in time, their problems will go away. Sometimes they do, but often sufferers don't realize that they need help until marriages have been lost, violations of the Uniform Code of Military Justice have been committed, or other life or career damage has been done.

The distinction between Orange Zone stress injury and Red Zone stress illness needs to be made by a clinical medical or mental health professional—not a unit leader, family member, or individual Marine or Sailor. The unit leader's responsibility is to recognize the possibility of Orange or Red Zone stress so that timely evaluation and treatment, if necessary, can take place. The presence of a Red Zone stress illness does not automatically render a Marine or Sailor unfit for duty or unfit for deployment. That is a judgment that must be made by the cognizant commander after the situation has been fully evaluated, taking into account all available information (see chap. 6). Since the wars in Iraq and Afghanistan began in 2001, many Marines and Sailors diagnosed and treated for PTSD in military medical facilities have recovered and been returned to full duty. Most of them have successfully finished their tours of duty and many are still serving.

# Traumatic Brain Injury

Traumatic brain injury (TBI) has been called the "signature injury" of the current wars in Iraq and Afghanistan. Improvements in vehicle and personal armor, along with advances in battlefield healthcare and medical evacuation, have made many injuries survivable that would have been fatal in past conflicts. Service members who survive improvised explosive device (IED) blasts or other attacks are now more likely to have injuries to the parts of the body least protected by armor—the head, face, and limbs.

The severity of a TBI is normally graded as mild, moderate, or severe based on the severity and persistence of alterations of consciousness in the immediate aftermath of the injury. (See app. B, *Traumatic Brain Injury Overview*, for details regarding how the severity of TBI is determined and for current guidelines on battlefield management of TBI.) There are several ways in which TBI, COSC, and OSC are related—

- TBI and stress injuries or stress illnesses, such as PTSD, often occur in the same individuals. The presence of one should alert unit leaders and caregivers to the possibility of another.
- Some of the symptoms of TBI, especially mild traumatic brain injury (mTBI), may be very similar or even identical to some of the symptoms of a traumatic stress injury or PTSD.
- There is increasing evidence that some of the same brain centers can be damaged by both a blast pressure wave and severe traumatic stress, which may explain some of the similarity in symptoms between mTBI and PTSD.
- An important tool in the initial treatment of both mTBI and stress injuries is rest.
- Both TBI and severe stress injuries, especially PTSD, involve literal damage to neurons in the brain, which tend to heal very slowly. The healing time for mTBI and PTSD may be similar.
- Deployment health assessments, such as the postdeployment health reassessment, screen for stress injuries and TBI.

Also important are the ways in which TBI and stress injuries differ from each other. Not all the symptoms of TBI, even mTBI, are exactly the same as symptoms of stress injuries. These two types of injuries can often be distinguished by their symptoms. The optimal medical treatments for TBI and stress injuries or illnesses differ significantly. While TBI may best be treated with either rest or retraining to relearn lost cognitive functions, stress disorders (such as PTSD, depression, and anxiety) have other very specific psychological and medication treatments.

Available measures for preventing TBIs and stress injuries are very different. The former are caused by either a blast or being struck on the head, while the latter are caused by intense or prolonged stress. Methods to protect Service members from blasts and stress are very different. Whereas Marines, Sailors, and family members can become more resilient and resistant to the effects of stress through training, social cohesion, and leadership, there are as yet no known methods of improving resistance to the damaging effects of blasts.

The frequent simultaneous occurrence and similarities between TBI and stress injuries or stress illnesses are reasons why unit leaders everywhere should be aware of current best practices for recognizing and managing them. Because of the important distinctions between TBI and stress injuries, the principles of COSC, OSC, and psychological health contained in this publication should not be construed to also apply to the prevention, recognition, or treatment of TBI.

# Core Leader Functions

The Navy-Marine Corps stress continuum model provides a framework for understanding and recognizing the spectrum of stress experiences and symptoms. This model, by itself, cannot improve the psychological health of Marines, Sailors, or family members or meet the two COSC and OSC objectives of preserving force readiness and maintaining individual health and well-being. In order to use the stress continuum model toward those ends, the Marine Corps and Navy have established the following five core leader functions, shown in figure 1-1 on page 1-16, for COSC and OSC across the stress continuum model:

- Strengthen.
- Mitigate.
- Identify.
- Treat.
- Reintegrate.

These core leader functions are briefly defined in the following paragraphs, but are also discussed in detail in chapters 2 through 6.

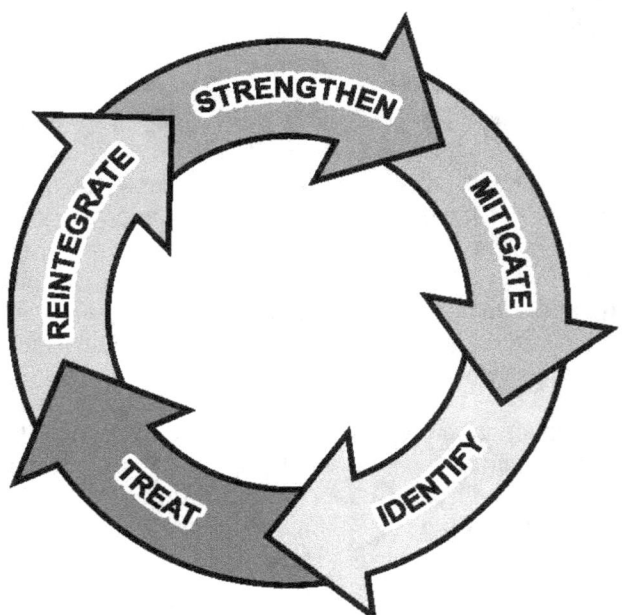

**Figure 1-1.** Five Core Functions of a Leader for COSC/OSC.

## Strengthen

Strengthening individuals, units, and families to enhance their resilience is the first core COSC and OSC function for military leaders. Individuals enter military service with a set of pre-existing strengths and vulnerabilities based on genetic makeup, prior life experiences, personality style, family supports, belief systems, and a host of other factors. Centuries of experience in military organizations and decades of scientific research have demonstrated that commanders of military units can do much to enhance the resilience of unit members and their families regardless of these pre-existing vulnerabilities. Activities available to commanders to strengthen their troops fall into three main categories—training, social cohesion, and leadership.

## Training

Tough, realistic training develops physical and mental strength and endurance, enhances warfighters' confidence in their abilities as individuals and as members of units to cope with the challenges they will face, and inoculates them to the stressors they will encounter. One challenge for unit leaders in strengthening their Marines and Sailors is to develop training that is tough and realistic enough to build resilience but does not inflict Orange Zone injuries.

## Social Cohesion

Social cohesion, defined broadly as mutual trust and support in a social group, is developed through shared experiences of accomplishment and overcoming adversity over time in a group with a stable membership. Social cohesion is a protective factor against the toxic effects of COS in both military units and families. Effective leaders know how to build cohesive units, given enough time and unit stability; however, the common challenge is to maintain unit cohesion in the face of frequent rotations into and out of the unit. These challenges include late joins, casualties, and combat replacements. Individual aug- mentees and members of Reserve Component units may be particularly disadvantaged regarding this important ingredient to resilience. Another challenge for unit leaders with respect to social cohesion is how to forge mutual trust and support among families left behind. Families are no less a part of the unit than the active duty Service members who deploy in cohesive units, but they often have much less opportunity to develop social cohesion with other families.

## Leadership

Although complex and multifaceted, leadership is an essential factor for the strengthening of unit members and families. Unit members are strengthened by leaders who teach and inspire them, keep them focused on mission essentials, instill confidence, and provide a model of ethical and moral behavior. Another crucial way in which leaders enhance the resilience of their unit members is by providing themselves as a resource of courage and fortitude on which unit members can draw during challenging times. The influence leaders have over their subordinates can also be detrimental if they too are experiencing Yellow, Orange, or Red Zone stress, unless their own stress is recognized and effectively managed.

## Mitigate

Since no Service member is immune to stress, regardless of strength or preparedness, the prevention of stress injuries and illnesses requires continuous monitoring and alleviation of the stressors to which individuals and units are exposed. Optimal mitigation of stress requires the balancing of competing priorities. There is the need to intentionally subject Service members to stress in order to train and toughen them and to accomplish assigned missions while deployed. At the same time, it is necessary to reduce or eliminate stressors that are not essential to training or mission accomplishment and ensure adequate sleep, rest, and restoration to allow recovery from stress between periods of challenge. Resilience, courage, and fortitude can be likened to leaky buckets that are constantly being drained by stress (see chap. 3). To keep them from running dry, these buckets must be frequently refilled through sleep, rest, recreation, and spiritual renewal. Continuing this metaphor, the leader function of mitigation is crucial to preventing more holes from being punched in these leaky buckets than are absolutely necessary.

Mitigation is a preventive activity aimed at keeping unit members in the Green "Ready" Zone when facing operational challenges and returning them to the Green Zone after Yellow Zone reactions. Specific tactics and procedures for unit leaders to mitigate COS are discussed in chapter 3.

## Identify

Since even the best preventive efforts cannot eliminate all stress reactions and injuries that might impact occupational functioning or health, effective COSC or OSC requires continuous monitoring of stressors and stress outcomes. Operational leaders must know the individuals in their units, including their specific strengths and weaknesses and the nature of the challenges they face both in the unit and in their home lives. Leaders must recognize when individuals' confidence in themselves, their peers, or leaders is shaken or when units have lost cohesion because of casualties, changes in leadership, or challenges to the unit. Most importantly, every unit leader must continuously monitor the stress zones of each unit member. It is particularly difficult for Service members to recognize their own stress reactions, injuries, and illnesses, especially while deployed to operational settings. The external focus of attention and the denial of comfort are necessary to thrive in an arduous environment and make it harder to recognize a stress problem in oneself. Stigma can also be an insurmountable barrier to admitting stress problems to someone else; therefore, the best and most reliable method of ensuring that everyone who needs help gets it is for small unit leaders to continually watch out for their subordinates and for peers to watch out for each other. Tools and procedures for unit leaders to identify stress reactions, injuries, and illnesses in Service members and family members are discussed in chapter 4.

## Treat

Available tools for the treatment of stress injuries and illnesses exist along a broad spectrum and include—

- Self-aid or buddy aid.
- Support from a small unit leader, chaplain, or corpsman.
- Definitive medical or psychological treatment.

Although some forms of treatment can only be delivered by trained medical or mental health providers (MHPs), many others require little special training and can be applied very effectively by anyone in almost any setting. Chapter 5 includes a detailed description of seven fundamental actions—the seven Cs of stress first aid—that can be taken by peers, family members, leaders, or caregivers to preserve life, to prevent further harm, and to promote healing from a stress reaction or injury. Stress first aid includes procedures for assessing the need for further care and coordinating with caregivers to ensure that help is received.

Regardless of what level or type of treatment is available and indicated for any given Marine or Sailor, the overall responsibility for ensuring that appropriate and timely care is delivered rests with unit leaders and their commanders. In order to increase the likelihood that care will be accepted by the individuals who need it, leaders must also attack stigma in all its forms within their units and organizations.

*Note:* To date, there is no well-established difference between an MHP and a mental health professional and the two terms are often used interchangeably. To be precise, though, the term provider can only be used for a mental health professional who is licensed and credentialed to practice independently, such as a psychiatrist, psychologist, licensed social worker, or licensed nurse practitioner. The term professional can be applied to anyone who has received specialized training, whether licensed or not, including psychiatric technicians, occupational therapists, and mental health counselors.

# Reintegrate

The normal course for a stress injury, as for a physical injury, is to heal over time, with most able to do so with or without treatment. Similarly, the normal course for a stress illness, especially if properly treated, is to improve significantly over time or completely remit. Hence, operational commanders face one final challenge in the management of Service members treated for stress injuries or illnesses—to continually monitor their fitness for duty, including worldwide deployment, and mentor them back to full duty as they recover. This vigilant monitoring is the challenge of reintegration. For stress casualties to be effectively reintegrated with their units, stigma must be continuously addressed and the confidence of the stress-injured Marine or Sailor, peers, and small unit leaders must be restored. This process may take months since recovery from a stress injury or illness is often a slow process. In those cases in which substantial recovery and return to full duty is not anticipated, the challenge for unit commanders is to assist Service members as they transition to civilian life and Veterans Administration care. Specific challenges for reintegration of Service members recovering from stress injuries or stress illnesses and techniques for meeting those challenges are discussed in chapter 6.

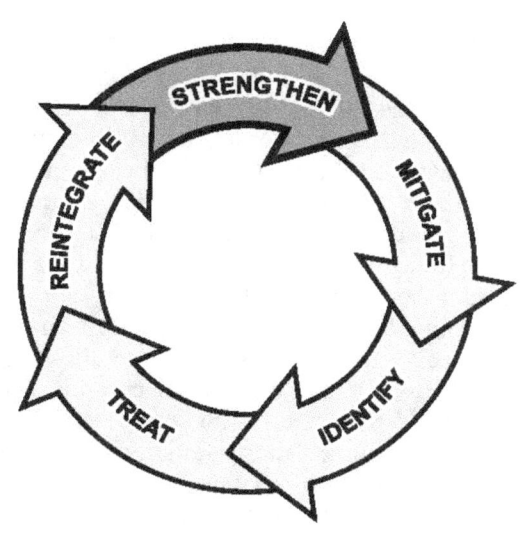

# 2

# STRENGTHEN: FIRST CORE FUNCTION FOR LEADERS

The first core COSC and OSC function for leaders is to strengthen their Marines and Sailors to enable them to successfully endure and master the stressors they will face during operational deployments. This first core function is also the most important for three reasons—

- Of all the actions leaders can take to manage the stress of their Marines and Sailors, strengthening them before exposure to COS has the greatest potential to actually prevent stress injuries and illnesses. An ounce of strengthening prevention is worth more than a pound of treatment and reintegration cure.
- Many of the actions leaders already take to prepare their Marines and Sailors for their operational duties can also, with only a slight change in focus, strengthen them against stress reactions, injuries, and illnesses. Strengthening for resilience and training for mission accomplishment are two strongly linked responsibilities of leaders.
- It is largely in the hands of unit leaders, regardless of the actions of medical, mental health, or religious ministry support personnel (see *Resilience: Responding to Challenges Across the Lifespan* for more information). To put it another way, if leaders don't strengthen their Marines and Sailors for resilience, usually no one else can or will.

# Strengthening for Resilience

Prior to an operational deployment, leaders need to know what specific physical and mental tasks their Marines or Sailors must perform for mission accomplishment in order to train them with the necessary skills that will strengthen them to meet expected challenges resiliently. Each specific mission poses unique challenges for mission-specific training and stressor-specific strengthening. Since it is impossible to list all the actions leaders might take to prepare their Marines or Sailors for every possible deployment challenge, a general model is presented in this chapter to prepare them for one specific type of stressor—direct life-threat or nearby experience of death. Life-threat stressors are among the most potentially toxic, leading in the worst cases to PTSD. Although the information that follows addresses strengthening to face life-threat stressors as one class of challenges, the principles conveyed apply to other classes of intense stressors as well, including loss and inner conflict.

## Effective and Resilient Response to a Life-Threat

A predictable sequence of mental events occurs in each individual during the first few moments after encountering a life-threat. Examples of life-threats that might initiate this sequence of events include nearly being killed by an IED blast, being ambushed and pinned down by small arms fire during ground combat, or witnessing the death of a shipmate in a fire below decks.

The sequence of mental events that happens after such an experience offers either optimal coping to counter the life-threat or less effective coping. The first outcome leads not only to effective performance but also to continued psychological wellness and increased self-confidence and resilience for future threat stressors. The latter may decrease resilience and lead to stress injury. The sequence of events discussed in the following paragraphs are only those that occur in the first moments after encountering a life-threat; subsequent responses by the individual and outcomes are determined by other factors and are not part of this discussion. The factors that determine which way this initial sequence of events goes—toward effective coping and resilience or ineffective coping and possible stress injury—are exactly the factors that need to be strengthened before exposure to a threat stressor in order to maximize resilience.

As shown in figure 2-1, the first event in this mind-body sequence occurs within a fraction of a second after the individual's senses perceive a threat in the environment—the response is entirely involuntary. An automatic internal alarm system in the brain and body triggers an immediate increase in heart rate, blood pressure, level of alertness, and other changes to prepare the body to take action. This activation in the body and brain can either contribute greatly to optimal functioning and the effective countering of an immediate threat or get in the way of effective coping if it is out of control. The brain's activation systems are based on the neuro-transmitters adrenaline and norepinephrine, which have an optimal range for effective performance. Like the engine in a car, the human brain and body perform best if they are kept within a certain operating range for coping responses to be effective.

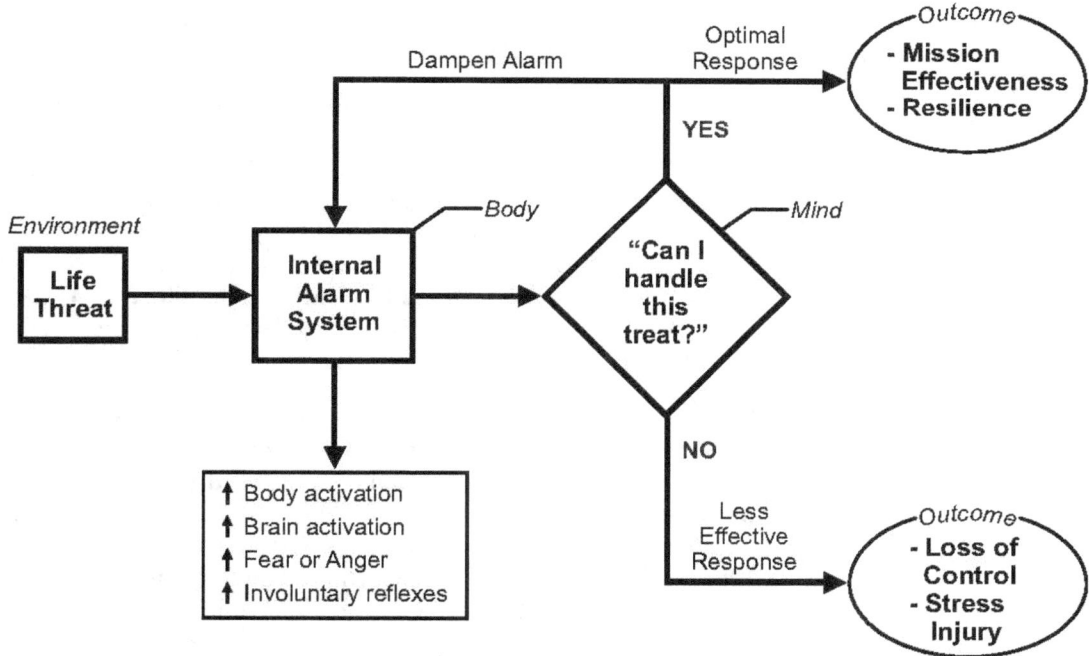

**Figure 2-1.** Initial Sequence of Events in Response to a Life Threat.

The internal alarm system also generates intense negative emotions, such as fear or anger, and triggers involuntary reflex behaviors, such as freezing, fleeing, or striking out blindly. These negative emotions and reflex behaviors must also be kept in check if the threat is to be countered most effectively.

The second event in this sequence, a moment later, is the mental process of deciding whether one believes oneself to be capable of mastering and surviving the threat. The question, "Can I handle this threat?" is not consciously deliberated; instead, it is an unconscious appraisal, occurring in a split second, of the threat situation and the internal and external resources available to deal with it. A snap judgment must be made based on the total of the individual's understanding, experience, and beliefs at that moment in time. Anything other than an immediate and emphatic, "Yes, I can handle this!" has the same effect as an immediate and equally emphatic, "No, I can't." Individuals may, however, later change their minds about their own capacities to conquer threats or to master challenges, but cannot easily talk themselves into really believing they can conquer threats if their initial appraisal of the situation is strongly negative.

The answer to the question, "Can I handle this threat?" has consequences of lasting importance for performance and well-being. If the answer is "yes," the individual is empowered to marshal available resources for effective action. Body and mind are mobilized to solve problems and to take action; behavior is focused and directed toward achieving success. If the threat is effectively neutralized, the individual is left with an enhanced sense of his or her own competence. Self-confidence increases as a result of having mastered one's own fear.

The mental power of really believing one can accomplish a task is well-known to military leaders. The more confident individuals are in themselves, peers, leaders, and equipment, the more likely they are to succeed. What is less well-known is the importance of a confidently positive answer to the question, "Can I handle this threat?" This confidence dampens the internal threat alarm system and bypasses distracting negative emotions or involuntary reflexes. A self-affirming "It's okay" or "I can do this" serves to calm the mind and body, leaving the individual open to clear thinking.

If the answer to the internal threat appraisal question is "No, I can't handle this," the opposite occurs. The internal alarm system is not dampened and the intensity of physical activation, negative emotions, or reflex behaviors all increase. Pushed beyond the optimal range, thinking may become unfocused and conscious control over negative emotions and behaviors may be lost. With this response, the ever-vigilant internal threat alarm system reappraises the situation to have become even more ominous because of these losses of control. After the threat has passed, if survived, the individual's sense of personal competence and self-confidence may be damaged as a result of having not effectively mastered the situation. Even worse, important control circuits in the brain may have been damaged by excessive and uncontrolled activation.

## Factors that Contribute to the Ability to Handle a Threat

Anything that empowers individuals in those initial seconds after encountering life-threats to say to themselves, "Yes, I can handle this," will make them not only more effective in the performance of their jobs but also more resilient to the potentially damaging effects of life-threat stressors. The following list identifies factors that leaders must strengthen in their Service members to ensure that they can respond in a positive manner when placed in a threat situation. These factors operate in four equally crucial domains—body, mind, spirit, and social, which includes unit, family, community, or other social support system. Strengthening actions must address all four domains to be optimally effective.

Body
- Necessary physical skills.
- Physical strength and endurance.
- Physical fitness and wellness.
- Healthy brain control systems for staying calm.

Mind
- Familiarity with the specific threat situation.
- Necessary mental skills.
- Self-knowledge and self-confidence.
- Psychological wellness.
- Willpower and fortitude.

Spirit
- Resources of fortitude from outside oneself.
- Belief in the rightness of mission and actions.
- Spiritual fitness.

<u>Social</u>
- Trust in peers, family, and the organization.
- Trust in leaders.
- Motivation to act on behalf of others.

## Strengthening the Body

Body factors necessary for effective coping and resilience include the requisite physical skills, strength, endurance, and other attributes needed to mount an effective response and to counter a particular threat. Physical wellness and fitness are critical for an optimal response to a threat. Conversely, the lack of physical wellness or fitness may significantly detract from an individual's ability and confidence. A further biological prerequisite for a positive threat response is the effective and normal functioning of the brain feedback circuits necessary for dampening the internal threat alarm as needed to keep negative emotions, involuntary reflexes, and body-brain activation under control. These brain systems are part of the essential infrastructure for positive coping, but they are also vulnerable to being reduced in effectiveness or even damaged by intense, long-lasting stress.

## Strengthening the Mind

Strengthening the mind for mounting an effective coping response and maintaining resilience begins with a familiarity with the specific threat situation encountered and the ability to recognize it as familiar. Familiarity may be the result of previous realistic training or similar operational experience. Unfamiliar situations may also be mastered by a Marine or Sailor who is able to generalize prior training or experience by adapting what was learned in the past to somewhat different situations in the present. The mental ability to generalize knowledge and skills and to adapt them to new situations requires intelligence, creativity, and self-confidence—all traits to be strengthened in Marines and Sailors to promote effective functioning and resilience.

A Marine or Sailor who possesses the necessary physical and mental skills to meet a challenge may be capable; however, to be truly strong, that Marine or Sailor must know he possesses those skills. Self-knowledge and self-confidence are keys to mental strength. Psychological wellness is crucial to using mental strength effectively and consistently.

The final contributors to mental strength—willpower and fortitude—are two aspects of courage. Fortitude is the ability to encounter danger or bear pain or adversity without faltering; whereas, willpower is the motivation to convert that mental strength into courageous behavior. These two crucial components of confidently handling a situation are also two of the least permanent or stable attributes. Knowledge and skill, once acquired, are not quickly lost, but willpower, fortitude, and courage are eroded by the wear and tear of continuous exposure to hardship and danger and may evaporate during an unexpected event. Willpower and fortitude are among the most important functions of leaders in military organizations.

## Strengthening the Spirit

Willpower and fortitude operate in the realm of the spirit as well as the mind. Maintaining and restoring these crucial ingredients of strength require individuals to refortify themselves with outside sources. No one possesses limitless resources of courage and perseverance, so everyone needs to augment their internal storehouse of fortitude by continually drawing upon sources beyond themselves that are revered and trusted, such as organizations, leaders, and the Divine. Believing one is on the right side of a conflict is also an important spiritual resilience factor for Marines and Sailors. Spiritual resilience is also based on firm trust in moral values and ethics. Deepening that trust and allowing nothing to damage it are crucial strengthening actions for leaders.

## Strengthening the Social Factors

Very much related to the spiritual aspects of resilience are the social factors in the unit or other social support system, such as family or community, which contribute to effective and resilient coping. Being surrounded by buddies or shipmates, who are known and trusted and with whom one has already mastered challenges and endured hardships, is a potent contributor to resilience. Likewise, being led by officers, noncommissioned officers (NCOs), or petty officers who have already earned trust through their competence and devotion to unit members is essential for effectiveness and resilience.

Other social systems outside the unit, such as families, friends, churches, or broader communities, exert a variable impact on resilience depending on the strength of attachment to these social systems by Marines or Sailors. Certainly, few stressors can sap the strength and willpower of a deployed Service member faster or more profoundly than an irresolvable family conflict or crisis back home.

# Strengthening Strategies

The strategies available to military leaders in the 21$^{st}$ century to strengthen their Marines, Sailors, or family members are much the same as those of the past. Changed and updated are the specific tactics, techniques, and technologies available to perform strengthening functions within each of three overall strategic categories—training, cohesion, and leadership. The remainder of this chapter describes each strategic category for strengthening and reviews general principles for understanding and devising tactics within each strategy. No attempt is made to provide an exhaustive list of tactics, techniques, or procedures for strengthening, since all leaders must develop their own specific strengthening tactics to meet the needs of their units and missions, taking into account the resources available to them.

## Training

Training, as the term is used in this publication, consists of all activities designed to instill necessary knowledge, skills, and attitudes (KSAs) in Marines or Sailors—both as individuals and as members of teams—to meet mission requirements and to remain resilient. Most relevant to the present discussion is not which specific KSAs are needed to meet mission requirements in any particular situation, but which KSAs are needed to strengthen Marines and Sailors against the stressors they will face so that they can become and remain resilient. Though most training meets both goals—mission and resilience—leaders must consider the resilience-building goal throughout their preparations for deployment and other operations to maximize strengthening training.

The KSAs needed for resilience building are the ones that empower a Marine or Sailor to make the snap judgment, "Yes, I can handle this," in the first moments of any situation and to keep making that positive judgment as the situation evolves. Crucial to this effort is the ability to know how to evaluate any possible training or educational activity for its impact on resilience and its ability to strengthen Marines and Sailors to endure and to master stress, as shown in figure 2-2. Appendix C, *Checklist for Evaluating Resilience Impact of Training*, provides a tool for leaders to evaluate planned training for its impact on the resilience of unit members. The basic principles for training to promote resilience are to—

- Make training as realistic as possible so that unit members will have few surprises during deployment. Intense surprise can be the worst enemy of psychological health.
- Make training tough enough to push unit members to develop new skills without making it so tough they fail to master training challenges or to experience stress injuries on the training range.
- Promote communication and trust both horizontally (peer to peer) and vertically (leader to subordinate) through shared hardships and programmed success.

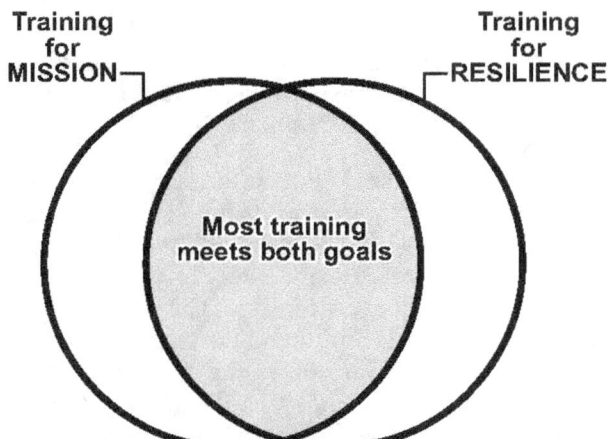

**Figure 2-2.** Overlap of Training for Mission Performance and Resilience.

## Cohesion

Social cohesion holds a group of people together, making them work together and achieve more as a unit than they would individually. Social cohesion is created in all social groups in much the same way, whether that group is a ground combat fire team, the crew of a ship, health care professionals taking care of acutely injured Marines and Sailors in a surgical hospital, or a

*A cohesive unit creates courage by reducing fear. The human brain codes social recognition, support, and attachement as safety.*

**Jonathan Shay**
*Odysseus in America: Combat Trauma and the Trials of Homecoming*

family in the United States. Cohesion in a unit or group develops gradually through the interaction of the following factors:

- Familiarity.
- Communication.
- Trust.
- Respect.
- Loyalty.
- Love.

Great military leaders know how to develop cohesion in their units. They know how to forge attachment, trust, loyalty, and love even in a group of strangers brought together for the first time to become a team. They know how to balance shared hardship with shared recreation and insurmountable challenges with unbelievable successes. The ability to develop and maintain unit cohesion has always been a valuable leadership skill because cohesive units are the most effective at accomplishing any mission assigned to them. Cohesive units function more as teams, while units lacking cohesion function more as a collection of individuals. Unit cohesion not only promotes effective performance, but also strengthens unit members to endure the toxic effects of operational stress and to be more resilient.

Unit cohesion helps Marines or Sailors respond to a threat situation with a positive, "Yes, I can handle this!" because in a cohesive unit, the "I" can be replaced with "we." In those first moments of response to a threat, members of cohesive units ask themselves, "Can *we* handle this threat?" This question is much easier to answer positively if unit members have learned through tough, realistic training or prior operational experience that their team can and will master tough challenges together. While surrounded by trusted peers, Marines or Sailors experience significantly less potentially harmful brain-body activation or intense negative emotion when their internal alarm systems are going off in response to an external life-threat. They are much less likely to lose cognitive focus or emotional or behavioral control. In cohesive units, unit members help each other refill their tanks of courage and fortitude as these become depleted under stress. Members of cohesive units help each other understand and make sense out of their challenges and sacrifices, so that their individual core values and other important beliefs are not damaged by intensely stressful events. Unit cohesion helps prevent stress injuries and illnesses.

Social cohesion can be thought of as being a form of social wellness or unit fitness. A healthy, cohesive unit is an important strengthening factor for unit members in ways that are similar to how unit members' personal physical and psychological health and fitness strengthen them as individuals. Since, just as with individuals, resilience for units is temporary and can be lost due to stress or other adverse events, physical and psychological fitness can only be developed and maintained through regular effort and attention. Just as physical or psychological health can be lost or diminished as a result of harmful events, unit cohesion can be lost or diminished as a result of specific social threats or challenges. To maintain healthy social cohesion, it is important for leaders to understand and recognize the following potential threats to the unit's cohesion and resilience of unit members:

- New accessions to the unit, especially just before deployment.
- Loss of unit members during deployment, whether as casualties or for other reasons.
- Turnover of unit members due to transfers soon after a deployment.
- Loss or turnover of leadership, especially just before or during a deployment.
- Events during deployment with unexpected or adverse outcomes, especially if there is a potential for blaming unit members or leaders for the outcomes.
- Any violations in the unit of ethics, rules of engagement, or core values.
- Hazing or other destructive behavior within the unit.
- The wear and tear of prolonged or repeated deployments, especially if there is insufficient time between deployments to recover fully.

Any of these threats to unit cohesion can result in a loss of trust, loyalty, communication, and respect among unit members. All can decrease the resilience of members of the unit.

## Leadership

The final strategy for strengthening—leadership—is the most fundamental of all because the other strategies for strengthening Marines and Sailors depend on it for their success. There can be no training or unit cohesion without the direct and continuous involvement of leaders, but leadership can also directly strengthen Marines and Sailors for resilience through discipline, example of fortitude, clear communication, and the promotion of ethics.

> *Leadership is the capacity to frame plans which will succeed and the faculty of persuading others to carry them out in the face of death.*
>
> **Lord Moran**
> *Anatomy of Courage*

## Instilling Discipline

The word "discipline" is often taken to mean "punishment" in common usage. In its original and broadest sense, discipline means instructing someone in a particular code of conduct by example and teaching the necessary self-control to live by that code. In this sense, learners are "disciples" who seek to mold themselves after their mentor, in whom the desired core values and code of conduct are clearly and consistently evident. Discipline is the means by which leaders at all levels communicate relentlessly to subordinates the entire set of KSAs they need to absorb and to master in order to answer every threat they will face with an immediate and resounding, "Yes, I can handle this!"

Because operational environments in the Navy and Marine Corps change over time, it is impossible for one single code of conduct or one single set of KSAs to apply to all Marines and Sailors in all possible situations. Core values apply to all, but all other aspects of a particular operational community's code of conduct must be specific to that community at that point in time; therefore, codes of conduct can only be taught by leaders who are true masters of their code. Toughness can only be taught by leaders perceived to be tough; thoughtfulness by the thoughtful; honesty by the honest. Few experiences for junior Marines or Sailors are more frustrating and destructive than to be disciplined by a leader who is viewed by subordinates as not living by the same code of conduct he expects of them.

## Being an Example of Fortitude

*One key characteristic of a great military leader is an ability to draw from the tremendous depths of fortitude within his own well, and in doing so he is fortifying his own men by permitting them to draw from his well.*

**Dave Grossman**
*On Killing*

The intangible qualities of willpower, fortitude, and courage to mental and spiritual strength are continually lost through the wear and tear of exposure to hardship and danger and through adverse events that surprise and overwhelm individuals or units.

How can Marines and Sailors replenish their fortitude? The ultimate resources for becoming refortified are those entities which are most powerfully cherished by the individual, such as "God, Country, and Corps," for many Marines, or "Ship and Shipmates" for seagoing Sailors. The difficulty with these ultimate wells of fortitude is that they can seem very remote and distant to Marines or Sailors who have seen their internal stores of courage drain away due to operational stress. In these instances, leaders, at their best, become the tangible, accessible, flesh-and-blood resources of fortitude and willpower that individual Marines and Sailors can draw upon in times of need. The same is true for line leaders, who draw some of their own fortitude from the larger military organization's traditions, honor, and values, and for chaplains, who draw some of their own fortitude from Divine sources. Regardless, the leaders who have the greatest potential for replenishing fortitude are those who have the most direct day-by-day and minute-to-minute contact with unit members.

## Communicating a Clear Vision

Leaders are communicators. Marines and Sailors thrive on clear communication regarding what outcomes are expected, how those outcomes will be achieved, and why they are worth achieving. This kind of vertical communication in units must operate in both directions to be most effective. The job of leaders is only half completed once they conceive a plan to achieve the ends desired and then communicate that plan to unit members. The second half of the job is to then hear from unit members whether they believe in this plan and see it as feasible or possible. Leadership to promote resilience requires both the capacity to tell subordinates what must be done and to listen to how those subordinates perceive and trust in the leader's plan. The reasons for a particular course of action and the meaning and relevance of the goals that are sought must be clearly communicated by leaders.

## Promoting Ethics and Protecting Core Values.

Resilience in the face of hardships and losses requires individuals to believe that what they are doing and what they have sacrificed has meaning and value—that they are contributing to a greater good. Clearly communicating the meaning and value of a unit's activities and challenges is one way a leader can promote this kind of crucial understanding and sense of purpose in unit members. Another fundamental way in which leaders can promote understanding and meaning is to ensure that all decisions made and all actions taken by unit members are consistent with organizational core values, the law of war, rules of engagement, and other ethical standards. In other words, it must *be* right. Leaders are the protectors and watchdogs of ethical decision-making and the core values of the organization. Deviations from ethical standards, if they occur, must be openly acknowledged and corrected before unit members mistakenly take such deviations as proof that the standards are not to be trusted or valued, but are merely hollow words.

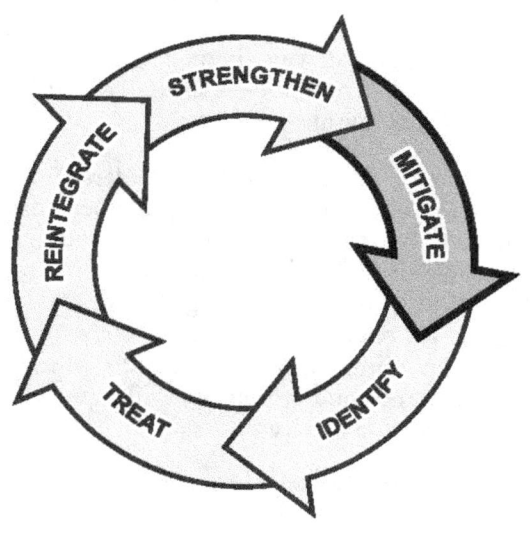

# MITIGATE: SECOND CORE FUNCTION FOR LEADERS

The second core COSC and OSC function for leaders is to mitigate the stress of their Marines and Sailors to keep them functioning optimally and to prevent the negative effects of stress reactions and stress injuries. The word "mitigate" literally means to reduce in force or intensity. Since no amount of strengthening will make anyone completely immune to stress, the crucial second step for leaders to maintain the psychological health of their units and family members is to reduce the force and intensity of the stressors they experience whenever possible.

In the ongoing battle between unit members and the stressors that continually attack their health and well-being—some in a slow siege over a long period of time, others all at once in a frontal assault—the first core function of strengthening can be thought of as the primary *defensive* weapon against stress and the second, the primary *offensive* weapon. Strengthening renders individuals less likely to be damaged by operational stressors. Mitigation attacks the stressors or lessens their impact on unit members and families. Both are essential to build and to maintain resilience. Strengthening and mitigation are a leader's tools for primary prevention.

The first and most obvious way to mitigate stress is to completely or partially eliminate the challenges that cause stress problems in Marines, Sailors, and family members. Eliminating stressors as a tactic for stress mitigation is analogous to preventing sunburn by keeping people out of direct sunlight. Eliminating stressors is the surest way to reduce the negative effects of stress, but it often isn't possible—especially in arduous and dangerous operational environments.

Fortunately, a second tactic is available to leaders for the mitigation of stress. The negative impacts of unavoidable stressors can be reduced in intensity by restoring the important biological, psychological, social, and spiritual resources that are depleted by those stressors. The "leaky bucket" analogy (see fig. 3-1) highlights the two targets for reducing the negative consequences of stress—minimizing or eliminating stressors to slow the depletion of available resources and storing up and replenishing resources that have been depleted by stress.

This chapter reviews categories of resources that can be crucial for resilience, including resources in the physical, mental, social, and spiritual domains. Common stressors that can drain resources are identified and leader actions for stress mitigation discussed. These actions include attacking potentially depleting stressors and

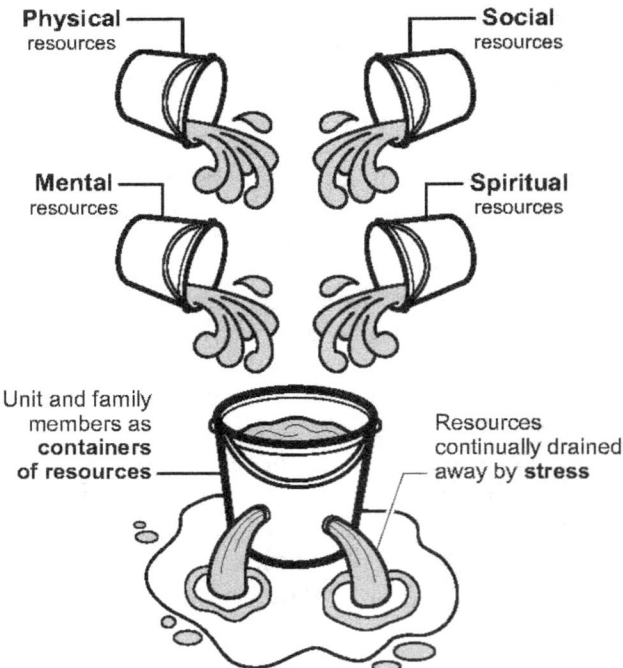

**Figure 3-1.** The "Leaky Bucket" Metaphor for Stress

directly replenishing resource stores in unit members. Appendix D, *Checklist for Preserving Resources to Mitigate Stress*, summarizes the content of this chapter and can be used as a leadership aid or teaching tool.

# Defining a Resource

Before reviewing specific categories of resources and methods for preserving and replenishing them, it is helpful to know what a resource for resilience is and how to recognize which particular resources are important for the resilience of specific unit and family members. As discussed in the research of Stevan E. Hobfoll in *Stress, Culture, and Community: The Psychology and Philosophy of Stress*, to master stress in their lives people depend on a very broad and diverse collection of both tangible and intangible assets.

A resource for resilience may be anything that people value, including things that are valued by nearly all people and others valued by only certain individuals. For example, almost everyone values health, money, prestige, meaningful work, and loving friends and family. Marines and Sailors all tend to value manifestations of honor, courage, and commitment in their lives. Married Marines and Sailors, especially those with children, tend to place great value on their homes and family lives, while young, single Service members tend to place greater value on socializing with peers. The personal pursuits that people find valuable, including hobbies, sports, and religious and social activities, vary significantly from person to person over the course of each person's life. Whatever each individual values and works to have and keep are resources for that person to cope resiliently with the challenges and hardships they face. To promote resilience, leaders must identify which particular resources are important to members of their units and then work to conserve them. The role of resources in stress and resilience can be summarized in the following points:

> *In the trenches, a man's willpower was his capital and he was always spending, so that wise and thrifty company officers watched the expenditure of every penny lest their men went backrupt. When their capital was done, they were finished.*
>
> **Lord Moran**
> *Anatomy of Courage*

- Everyone needs resources to cope with stress effectively and to stay well.
- Resources can be physical, mental, emotional, social, or spiritual.
- Life challenges are stressful. They drain, deplete, or threaten to deplete needed resources in one way or another.

- Stress can be reduced by either attacking the stressors that deplete needed resources, by replenishing the stores of specific resources drained away by stress, or both.
- Because they tend to be tough and highly motivated, Marines and Sailors can "run on empty" longer than most people, but no one can do it indefinitely.
- Like engines forced to run without lubrication, people forced to operate with too few resources are at great risk for stress injuries and illnesses.
- Resources are also crucial for recovering from stress injuries, although the resources needed for healing may be different from those previously valued.

# Conserving Physical Resources

*Willpower, determination, mental poise, and muscle control all march hand-in-hand with the general health and well-being of the man.*

**S.L.A. Marshall**
WWII Army
Combat Historian
*Men Against Fire: The Problem of Battle Command*

Two categories of physical resources are important for the resilience of Marines, Sailors, and family members—biological resources that are fundamental for the healthy functioning of the body and brain and environmental resources that affect individual resilience less directly through their impact on mental well-being. Some ways to conserve physical health and well-being include the following:

- Know the Marines and Sailors in the command.
- Monitor Marines and Sailors closely for signs of injury or illness.
- Take care of health problems early.
- Use protective equipment.
- Practice safety procedures.
- Model rational sleep discipline.
- Allow adequate rest and down time.
- Encourage and reward physical fitness.
- Teach and encourage optimal nutrition.
- Teach hygiene, first aid, and self- and buddy care.
- Limit exposure to extremes of weather.

## Physical Health and Well-Being

The basic essential personal resources for effective performance and resilience are those contributing to physical health and well-being. Without fit, healthy, and well-functioning bodies, even the most highly motivated Marines and Sailors may not be able to convert their willpower into effective action or successfully endure the physical or mental hardships they will encounter. Because the mind is firmly rooted in the electrochemical activity of the brain, physical health is a prerequisite for effective mental function, including accurately assessing challenging situations, developing rational plans to master them, and remaining calm and focused as those plans are implemented.

Many of the risks to the physical health and well-being of Marines and Sailors deployed to operational environments are obvious. Depending on the mission and location, the greatest risks to physical health may be incoming projectiles, IED blasts, accidents, falls, fires, communicable diseases, foodborne bacteria, heat, or insect bites. Each of these risks can be reduced through the application of specific countermeasures already developed to meet them. Other risks to the physical health of Marines and Sailors and the physical resources they deplete are less obvious, even though their potential impacts on unit members' functioning and resilience are no less great. The following subparagraphs discuss five less obvious, but no less crucial, physical health resources and the hazards that may deplete them.

## Sleep

Most people require a minimum of 6 to 8 hours of sleep each day to replenish the chemicals in their brains and bodies needed for clear-headed thinking, steady emotions, optimal immune system functioning, and resilience to stress. With training and experience, Marines and Sailors can learn to not feel tired after only 4 hours sleep, but they cannot be trained to function at their best or stay mentally and physically well on so little sleep for more than a few days. After being deprived of sleep, whether gradually over many days or weeks or all at once, Marines and Sailors suffer from decreased clarity of thought, slowed recall of information, diminished ability to rationally solve problems, decreased emotional calmness in life-threatening situations and a loss of overall resilience to stress and immunity to illness. One indicator of the potentially serious impact of sleep loss on operational performance was the experience by many sleep-deprived ground combat troops participating in the initial invasion of Iraq in 2003. Many reported experiencing repeated visual hallucinations, including seeing shapes and shadows moving across the desert landscape that were hard to distinguish from real enemy forces.

> *For most people, getting only 4 hours of sleep per day for a week causes as great loss of mental acuity as staying up for 36 hours straight.*
>
> **Van Dongen, Maislin, Mullington, Dinges**
> *Sleep* Magazine

To prevent the insidious adverse effects of sleep deprivation, sleep regimens must be enforced and make-up sleep must be ensured soon after periods of unavoidable sleep deprivation. Leaders must continuously challenge misconceptions among their Marines and Sailors about sleep and leaders must attack existing military cultural norms that place a high value on the apparent ability to function without sleep. In this regard, leaders' most powerful tools for positive change are their own consistent example of sleep discipline and their habit of rewarding subordinates who excel at their jobs in spite of spending 6 to 8 hours each day asleep.

## Physical Fitness

The importance of physical strength and endurance for mission accomplishment is well-known to Marines and Sailors operating in physically demanding specialties, such as those involving ground combat. Less well-known is the crucial role physical fitness plays in optimal mental performance and stress resilience for all Service members, even those in less physically demanding roles. Physically fit Marines and Sailors tend to have lower heart rates and lower risks for traumatic stress injury in life-threatening situations than those who are less fit. Marines and Sailors who are physically fit are better able to sustain mental focus and cognitive readiness in challenging technical roles in spite of the fatigue of long and frequent watches or prolonged boredom. Research has shown that physically fit individuals are more resilient to the resource-depleting effects of various stressors, as if their resource "buckets" were simply larger than those of other, less fit individuals.

Physical exercise and fitness also enhance resilience through the psychological benefits of increased self-confidence and self-esteem and the biological effects of reduced levels of toxic stress chemicals and increased levels of naturally occurring antidepressants and antianxiety hormones in the body. High levels of these natural stress-buffering chemicals in response to a stressor are a key biological discriminator between highly trained, elite combat forces and other, less well-trained or resilient troops.

The higher their stress levels, the more all Marines and Sailors, regardless of military occupational specialty, need to engage in regular, sustained physical exercise. Leaders should not only model the challenging task of fitting time for physical exercise and training into a full schedule, but recognize and reward physical fitness efforts among their unit members as contributing to both physical and mental readiness.

## Core Body Temperature

The human body and brain function best when the core body temperature is kept in the range of 96.8 to 100.4 degrees

Fahrenheit. At temperatures above or below this range many mental functions quickly deteriorate, including motivation, mental alertness, speed and accuracy of information recall, and time to react to a threat. Healthy bodies can regulate their core temperatures within the normal range only if not subjected to excessive heat gain or loss from the environment. Extremes of ambient heat or cold, radiation from sunlight or other sources, and high humidity can all accelerate heat absorption or loss, pushing the core body temperature outside its healthy operating range. Marines and Sailors may not be aware of or able to tell anyone about decrements in performance or resilience due to changes in their core body temperatures. Core body temperatures, like other physical resources, must be closely monitored and tightly conserved by leaders.

## Nutrition

Fuels and other necessary chemical resources in the body and brain are manufactured in the body mostly from raw materials contained in the diet. Fortunately, the ability of the body to manufacture these crucial resources is not very sensitive to short-term changes in the amount or types of foods ingested. However, prolonged restriction of the intake of important raw materials can lead to severe changes in health and resilience. Prolonged hunger also raises baseline levels of physiological activation, causing higher pulses and blood pressures even at rest. This places food-deprived Marines and Sailors at greater risk for deterioration of mental performance and possible stress injury during any additional exertion or stress. Food is a resilience resource that should be treated with the same respect as all other resources for health and well-being.

## Stigma of Admitting to Physical Injury or Illness

The stigma associated with mental health problems is well recognized. Members of all Services have reported a reluctance to seek help for stress or mental health problems for fear of being branded as weak by their peers and superiors. Less well-known, but of equal importance, is the stigma in certain segments of the military associated with seeking help even for a *physical* health problem, especially if it is an injury or illness not caused by direct enemy action. Particularly in ground combat communities in which toughness and stoicism are highly prized, Marines and Sailors may suffer through entire deployments with mild to moderate physical health problems they are unwilling to report to their leaders or medical personnel for fear of being seen as less tough or of being removed from their duties and units. Leaders at all levels must remain vigilant for unreported physical health problems that may get much worse before finally receiving treatment after deployments are over. They must create unit cultures that value self-care and buddy care to maintain readiness whenever needed.

## Personal Possessions and Space

Young men and women do not enlist or seek commissioning in the Marine Corps or Navy because they want to get rich and live in luxury. Marines and Sailors know they will neither become wealthy serving their country, nor will their opportunities for increased income in the future match those of their civilian peers. These realities do not diminish the importance of a continual inflow of sufficient monetary resources to pay the bills, live in a comfortable house, own one or two working vehicles, put nutritious food on the table, and dream of a better life in the future. Money, personal possessions, and personal space all serve as crucial resources for resilience in a number of ways, all of which are important for unit leaders to understand.

While considering the importance of personal possessions to individual resilience, it is helpful to keep in mind the basic principle common to all resources for resilience—losing a particular resource or even being threatened with the loss of that resource has a greater negative impact on well-being and resilience than never having had that resource in the first place. Each loss of resources—even a small loss—takes a big bite out of resilience.

How can a Marine or Sailor suffer a loss of personal possessions? The number one cause of loss of personal possessions by Service members and families is a loss of personal income needed to acquire, maintain, and replace valued personal possessions. Personal possessions can also be lost due to accident or theft. Access to personal possessions can easily be lost due to deployments, transfers, temporary duty assignments, individual augmentation, and many other situations that separate Marines and Sailors from the possessions they value. Personal space, as a resource for resilience, may be nearly nonexistent in certain close-quarter operational situations. It can also be lost due to operational movement of the unit, damage to living quarters, or infringement on personal space by others. The following are a few of the ways in which personal possessions and personal space contribute to personal resilience.

## Income as a Determinant of Socioeconomic Status

Along with one's level of educational attainment and occupation, income level is a primary determinant of socioeconomic status—the unofficial system of social standing in our country that assigns relative ranks to individuals and families based on achievements and potential to contribute to the common good. To some extent, everyone needs to feel respected, admired, and esteemed by others in society. Social standing based on socioeconomic status can be a powerful buttress to individuals' resilience to stress. Conversely, individuals who have lost social standing because of loss of income, loss of rank, change to a less prestigious job, or conviction of a crime have diminished resilience to other life stressors. Some common reasons for the loss of personal income include the following:

- Marine or Sailor unable to work a second or third job while deployed.
- Spouse unable to work as much while Service member is deployed due to child care needs.
- Spouse or child illness or injury.
- Family breakup.
- Family transfer to an area where employment for spouse is unavailable.
- Reduction in rank.
- Fines or forfeiture of pay.
- Excessive indebtedness.
- Poor financial management.
- Civilian legal fines and fees.

## Money as a Universal Problem Solver

Many of the threats to well-being faced by individuals and families require monetary solutions. Health problems may require expensive treatments, legal problems often cannot be resolved until legal fees and fines are paid, education and training to raise standards of living are usually not free, and lost or destroyed personal possessions cannot be replaced without money. Hence, individuals with lower levels of personal income have fewer resources to solve life's problems.

## Money and Vehicles as Necessary for Independence

Individuals and families who lack financial resources to solve their own problems or to neutralize threats to their personal well-being must often depend on other individuals or organizations for financial assistance. Likewise, individuals who do not possess personal vehicles, especially in areas where public transportation is poor, may have to beg a ride from someone else every time they need to get somewhere. Some adults in our society, especially young adults, may not suffer a loss of self-esteem for needing to depend on the generosity of others to solve their life problems, but most mature adults in our society dread dependency on others because of its negative impact on self-concept and self-respect. Money and possessions contribute to self-esteem and well-being to the extent they make independence and self-reliance possible.

## Possessions as Familiar Features of Environment

People differ somewhat in the extent to which they become emotionally attached to the inanimate objects they possess or in which types of objects they find value and meaning. Furthermore, the Spartan warrior ethos—the denial of physical comfort to enhance physical and moral strength and courage—found in Marine and Navy cultures discourages reliance on personal possessions for coping with stress and maintaining well-being. Nevertheless, everyone has attachments to personal objects that offer them comfort during times of stress, such as pictures, letters, books, music, movies, laptop computers, digital music players, and cameras. Everyone also derives comfort from being surrounded by familiar sights, sounds, smells, and tactile sensations.

Like other resources, the impact of personal possessions on resilience and well-being becomes most relevant when possessions are lost or when events threaten their loss. The trauma individuals/families experience in the wake of a hurricane, for example, may be exclusively due to the loss of important possessions, such as homes, vehicles, furniture, clothing, and irreplaceable articles of high emotional significance. People who lose valued objects may go through a mourning process indistinguishable from the process of grieving the death of a loved one.

## Personal Space as a Safe Retreat

Marines, Sailors, and family members also strive to carve out and to retain private, personal spaces in which to experience comfort and safety, to retreat from conflict and contact with others when desired, and to rest. Personal space is an important buffer zone for stress and its absence, as occurs in overcrowded slums and concentration camps, has repeatedly been shown to increase the risk of destructive interpersonal aggression, other forms of misconduct, and mental and physical health problems. Personal space is a scarce resource in operational environments of all kinds and available space is seldom distributed evenly among all unit members. Deployed Marines and Sailors should be allocated as much privacy as possible for berthing and personal spaces should be protected. Some ways to conserve personal possessions and space include the following:

| Research has shown that humans routinely experience more stress, disease, aggression, and early mortality as they are crowded together into smaller spaces. |
|---|

- Helping Marines, Sailors, and family members plan for unexpected losses of income.
- Keeping unit and family members informed of deployment schedules as early as possible.
- Teaching financial management.
- Ensuring continuous access to important personal possessions to the extent operationally feasible.
- Creating a unit culture of respect for personal possessions and space.
- Allowing part-time employment during off-hours, if warranted.
- Allocating maximum space for living quarters.

# Conserving Mental and Emotional Resources

Mental and emotional resources can be divided into three partially overlapping categories—safety and security, morale, and pride and self-esteem. Resources in these three categories are all intangible internal states of thought and feeling. Fortunately, leader actions to conserve these mental and emotional resources are more tangible and include very specific actions to influence either the ways in which Marines and Sailors experience their environment or the nature and content of vertical and horizontal interactions within the unit.

## Safety and Security

The feeling of security that comes from believing one is physically safe is a basic human need and a crucial resource for resilience. In his famous "Hierarchy of Needs," the American psychologist Abraham Maslow (see *A Theory of Human Motivation*) ranked safety and security as second only to life-sustaining needs, such as air, water, and food, in their importance for personal well-being (see fig. 3-2). Marines and Sailors participating in military operations are not much different from civilians in their biologically-rooted need to feel safe and secure, regardless of how accustomed they may have become to living and working in dangerous environments or how courageously they perform their duties in the shadow of death and destruction. They have this need because physical courage in the face of danger is partly grounded in the ability to banish from conscious awareness any thoughts, feelings, or images pertaining to death or injury, even though these may be imminent. Some stressors that can erode feelings of safety and security include the following:

- Life-threatening situations of all kinds.
- Unexpected threats to life, such as ambushes or concealed IED blasts.
- Death or serious injuries to peers, especially when witnessed.
- Witnessing the aftermath of death up close.
- Handling bodies and body parts.
- Taking care of the dying or seriously injured.
- Being relegated to a passive, defensive position while one's life is being threatened.
- Friendly fire incidents.

Effective functioning and resilience amid danger depend on a positive answer to the question, "Can I handle this threat?" For most individuals in most situations, "Yes, I can handle this!" is equivalent to saying, "Not only can I do what is needed to master this challenge, but I can and *will* survive it."

Subjective safety and security can be enhanced prior to operational deployment through leader actions for strengthening, including those focused on training, unit cohesion, or leadership. During deployments or training missions that mimic deployments, leaders can enhance their unit members' feelings of security by limiting close-up exposure to experiences of death and its aftermath whenever possible. This limitation reduces the negative impact on these feelings of security when such exposure cannot be avoided, increases real or perceived safety and security, and quickly restores lost confidence in self, peers, leaders, equipment, or mission.

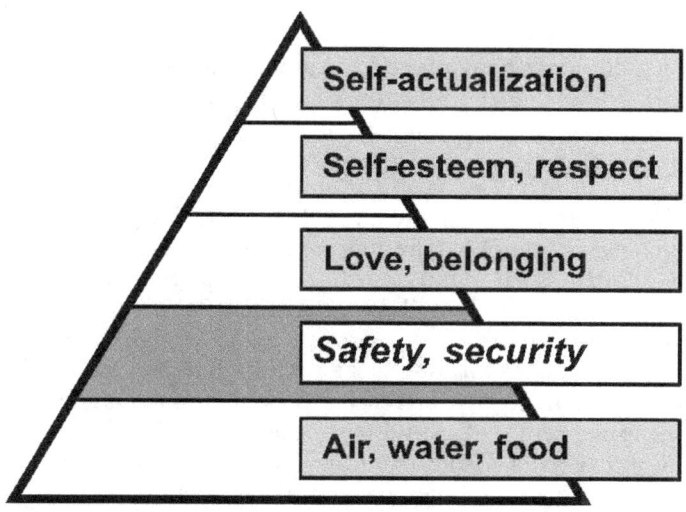

**Figure 3-2.** Maslow's Hierarchy of Needs.

## Minimize Close-Up Exposure to Death and its Aftermath

Experiencing the nearby sights, sounds, and smells of death is sometimes unavoidable in military operations. Individuals vary considerably in their vulnerability to losing their own feelings of safety and security by experiencing someone else's death. Any time unit members watch someone die, handle body parts, or witness scenes of carnage, their personal feelings of safety can be eroded. This risk is greatest for unit members who personally knew the deceased or closely identified with them because of similarities in age, gender, appearance, or some other factor. The more Service members perceive the dead or dying as similar to themselves, the harder it is for Marines and Sailors to maintain their own feelings of safety and security in the presence of others' very obvious mortality. Also, the greater their overall stress level, the more vulnerable Marines and Sailors are to being damaged by a close-up exposure to death. Since any close-up experience of death can seriously undermine necessary feelings of safety and security, it makes sense to limit all such exposures to the extent operationally feasible. The following practices help limit such exposure:

- Cover the dead, especially their hands and faces.
- Discourage gawking, even though it is human nature to want to witness death up close.
- Don't allow unit members to examine the personal effects of deceased personnel, unless their jobs require it.

## Prepare for the Unexpected

Surprise during a life-threatening situation is the greatest enemy of psychological health. The more unexpected a threat to life is, the more intensely it will trigger the brain's internal alarm system and the more likely it will be to generate overwhelming fear. Unanticipated attacks or accidents cause high degrees of physiological activation, such as a very high heart rate and blood pressure, which greatly increases the risk for a loss of mental sharpness and self-control and for possible stress injury. Preparing for the unexpected to the extent possible reduces the impact of life-threatening experiences on necessary feelings of safety and security. For example, if a scene of carnage must be viewed by members of a unit, one technique is to have one person survey the scene first and describe it in vivid detail to other unit members before they experience it.

## Take Action

> *Action is the great steadying force. It helps clear the brain.*
>
> **S.L.A. Marshall**
> WWII Army
> Combat Historian
> *Men Against Fire: The Problem of Battle Command*

Being stuck in a passive, helpless position during a time of life-threat adds significantly to stress and increases the likelihood of traumatic stress injuries. Marines and Sailors should get physically mobilized and take action—any action—to increase their feelings of mastery, confidence, and safety. Spouses and children at home may also find their roles—as passive, helpless observers—particularly challenging, so leading families to take action to increase their feelings of mastery and security is also crucial for their resilience.

## Attend to Physical Safety as Much as Possible

Even small efforts to improve the physical safety and security of the unit's position or to defend against known threats and hazards may pay large dividends in an enhanced ability of Marines and Sailors to maintain their confidence in their security in spite of immediate dangers.

## Use After Action Reviews after Casualty Events to Restore Confidence

Appendix E, *The After Action Review*, details procedures for using after action reviews (AARs) in small units as a tool for restoring mental, emotional, and social resources. The AARs should be conducted with Marines and Sailors in small groups led by their unit leaders with no outsiders present and with open and honest communication encouraged. These reviews can be helpful after any operational or training event in which there were casualties, accidents, or mistakes. The leader's resilience-related goal in conducting an AAR following a life-threatening event is to anticipate and restore lost confidence in self, peers, leaders, equipment, and mission in order to increase feelings of safety and security in the unit. If mistakes were made, unit members need to know that the unit learned from its mistakes so they won't be repeated. If unit members' conceptions of what happened are distorted by rumors and misinformation, those misconceptions must be corrected. The times during which honest discussions about recent events are most crucial for restoring lost confidence and security in a unit are precisely the times when such discussions will be very hard for leaders to facilitate. Avoiding talking about events that have damaged unit member trust does nothing to restore it and may erode trust even further.

*The most significant determinant of the effectiveness of unit after action reviews was the exclusion of outsiders from unit discussions.*

**Keinan, Keren**
Presentation at the September 2007 Military Psychology Center Conference, Tel Aviv, Israel.

## Morale

According to US Army Training and Doctrine Command Pamphlet 525-3-7-01, *The US Army Study of the Human Dimension in the Future 2015-2024*, morale may be defined as an individual's level of motivation, commitment, and enthusiasm for accomplishing unit mission objectives under stressful conditions. Although high morale has been considered a significant feature of effective units and a vital component of individual resilience, morale is difficult to quantify or to control. More like the weather than climate, morale can change rapidly and profoundly from moment to moment and day to day; nevertheless, morale is an important resource for resilience that leaders must work to monitor and to maintain in their units. The following paragraphs discuss actions leaders can take to enhance morale. Some stressors that can decrease individual or unit morale include the following:

- Long or extended deployments.
- Deployments of uncertain length.
- Closely repeated deployments.
- Turnover of key leaders.
- Abusive or unsupportive leadership.
- Boredom or a lack of accomplishment.
- Loss of confidence in self, peers, leaders, equipment, or mission.
- Breakdown of two-way communication in unit.
- Loss of means to communicate with families.
- Breakdown of discipline.
- Inconsistent rewards for accomplishment or consequences for misconduct.

## Listen to Marines and Sailors

Leaders who excel at influencing their Marines and Sailors through the force of their personalities and the respect they command in their units are sometimes less effective at just spending time with and listening to their unit members; listening is as vital a component of effective leadership as telling. The simple act of listening with genuine interest to Marines and Sailors as they talk about whatever is important to them can contribute enormously to morale. Personal time with a respected leader is seldom forgotten by a unit member.

During times of great stress there may be little else a leader can do to improve individual morale. Marines or Sailors who are wounded, ill, or experiencing crises in their personal lives may derive lasting benefit from a leader spending a few moments with them with no other objective than to understand how they feel and to let them know they are appreciated.

## Keep Unit Members Informed

Unit and family members who aren't reliably informed of unit schedules and anticipated missions fill the void in their knowledge with imagination and rumor, which are seldom constructive to morale. The less information members receive, the more helpless, passive, and less respected by their leaders they feel. Bad news never gets better over time and everyone benefits from advance warning to avoid surprises.

## Set and Achieve Realistic Unit Goals

Marines and Sailors don't need big victories to feel that their efforts and sacrifices are justified, but their morale depends on the continuous achievement of worthwhile goals. They need to continuously set unit goals that are challenging but achievable, communicate these goals to unit and family members, and acknowledge success when these goals are acheived.

## Minimize the Length of Deployments and Underway Periods

The length of deployments is also seldom under the control of unit leaders, but, if choices are possible, shorter is better than longer for psychological health. Longer deployments strain morale, marriages, and resilience. If deployments must be extended, losses of morale may be minimized just by keeping unit members informed of the reasons for the extension and the purposes served by their continued deployment.

## Maximize Dwell Time Between Deployments

Unit leaders usually have control over neither the dwell time available to unit and family members between deployments, nor the amounts and types of training required to prepare the unit for the next deployment. To the extent dwell time is flexible, it is important to keep in mind how critical that time is to unit members, especially those with families. Everyone needs a period of reduced stress after a challenging deployment to recover from deployment stressors and to solve problems that arose during deployment.

# Pride and Self-Esteem

Pride and self-esteem stem from the value individuals place in themselves and the worth they believe they have as individual human beings and as members of various organizations, including the military, their families, and their faith communities. Self-esteem consists of many factors from the past and present. Some of these factors are objective and rational, based on the individual's real merits and accomplishments, while others are more subjective and are based on either inflated or deflated perceptions about oneself. Regardless of what comprises an individual's self-concept and self-worth, these appraisals of self are powerful determinants of resilience. Marines and Sailors who exhibit high self-esteem and strong personal pride are more likely to believe that every challenge they face is within their ability to master. Conversely, individuals with very low self-esteem may lack confidence that they can master a difficult challenge; moreover, they may even see themselves as not worthy of being successful or even surviving a life-threat. Some stressors that can damage pride and self-esteem include the following:

- Personal failures or perceived failures.
- Unit failures or perceived failures.
- Mistakes and accidents.
- Misconduct.
- Being shunned by peers.
- Being criticized in public by leaders.
- Self-blame (guilt) for failing to protect a peer or leader from death or injury.
- Self-blame (shame) for failing to perform as expected because of physical or stress injury.

Military leaders know that individuals with high levels of self-esteem are more resilient and capable, especially if their pride and self-esteem are based in large measure on their belonging to a military unit with a high collective pride and *esprit de corps*. Effective military leaders are highly skilled at developing collective and individual pride in units and unit members. The strengthening leader actions reviewed in the last chapter all contribute to the resilience resource of positive self-esteem and pride in Marines and Sailors prior to deployment. To maintain high levels of pride and self-esteem during challenging and arduous operational deployments, additional leader actions are needed to mitigate the negative impacts on unit members' self-esteem because of stressful events and to restore and repair self-esteem that has been damaged by those events. The following paragraphs discuss three such leader actions.

## Teach Honorable
## Correction of Mistakes and Failures

Marines and Sailors may need to be taught how to honestly acknowledge their mistakes and failures and then to correct them without losing their honor and self-respect. Second chances to succeed, sometimes after additional training, can restore damaged self-esteem. Sometimes individuals need to be mentored to atone for their mistakes or failures and to make amends to those who were harmed before they can recover their self-esteem. The old maxim, "praise in public, criticize in private," applies here. The example leaders set by their own integrity, honest self-appraisals, and ability to maintain their personal honor in spite of their human failings can be powerful teaching tools.

## Mentor Those Who Commit Misconduct to Restore Their Honor

Even Marines and Sailors who commit misconduct and are facing incarceration or disciplinary or administrative discharges deserve respect for having served their God, Country, and Corps or Ship and Shipmates. Mentor them to make amends for their misconduct whenever possible and to restore their honor in spite of what they did. Other unit members observe how offenders are treated, learning from this how deeply the organization and its leaders are committed to those from whom unfaltering commitment is expected. Those Marines and Sailors who are forgiven for their misconduct after repaying what they owe may serve even more honorably in the future.

## Anticipate and Correct Exaggerated Self-Blame Through After Action Reviews and One-on-One Counseling

Accidents, casualties, and other negative outcomes are seldom the responsibility of just one person; however, Marines and Sailors who participate in such incidents sometimes blame themselves exclusively for what happened. Such guilt can be wildly exaggerated, not based on the facts of the incident, and corrosive to their self-esteem and psychological health. Anticipate who in the unit might be blaming themselves excessively and correct exaggerated self-blame during individual counseling or small unit AARs, as described in appendix C.

If blame exists, it should be apportioned fairly and shared by all who contributed to the outcome. Often, all that is needed to correct exaggerated self-blame is to point out how unrealistic, unfair, and unproductive it is and how, if roles were reversed, they wouldn't blame another unit member for what happened. Other influential leaders, such as chaplains, medical officers, and corpsmen, can also help reduce inappropriate and exaggerated self-blame, but unit leaders who are respected and trusted by their Marines and Sailors can be uniquely effective in this regard because of their credibility.

# Conserving Social Resources

Individuals vary greatly in the degree to which they rely on social supports to master the stressors they face and on which particular relationships they depend for their well-being. Even the most isolated loner needs social resources, especially from their two most important sources—peer support within the unit and family support from spouse, children, parents, siblings, and members of the extended family. Some stressors that can corrode unit cohesion and peer support include the following:

- Loss of unit members due to casualties, transfers, or separations.
- Gain of new unit members as transfers or replacements.
- Turnover of leadership, especially during, just before, or after a deployment.
- Deaths or injuries in the unit.
- Violations of ethics or rules by unit members, especially if unaddressed by unit leaders.
- Hazing.
- Breakdowns of or obstacles to horizontal (peer-to-peer) communication.

## Peer Support

Unit cohesion, defined as a high degree of communication, trust, and support among members of a unit, is a vital strengthening factor to be developed by unit leaders prior to deployment. During deployment, unit cohesion is crucial to maintaining resilience among unit members, especially when the unit has taken casualties, been exposed to life-threatening stressors, or performed difficult missions under arduous conditions. The greater the stress experienced by a deployed unit, the closer its members become to one another and the more they depend on each other for their psychological health and well-being.

Vital unit cohesion can be damaged by a number of stressors, including casualties, changes in unit composition, and events that cause a breakdown in communication or trust. To conserve peer support as a resource for resilience, leaders must continually monitor the level of cohesion in their units, recognize and neutralize threats to that cohesion, and augment peer support through ongoing team-building activities. Like the chain that is only as strong as its weakest link, unit cohesion may be only as strong as that surrounding the least well-integrated, supported, and trusted unit member. The following are leader actions to conserve peer support throughout training missions and operational deployments as a resource for resilience.

## Incorporate New Unit Members Quickly

Like weak links in a chain, new accessions to operational units can be detriments to unit effectiveness and cohesion as well as to their own safety and well-being, especially if they join immediately before or during a deployment. Until they are tested and can prove their abilities and their loyalty to other unit members, new additions to a unit may detract from the confidence and sense of security of all who must depend on them. Similarly, until other unit members establish feelings of loyalty toward new additions to the unit, their feelings of safety and security will also remain low. Studies of the "new guy" phenomenon during the Vietnam War confirmed that new accessions to combat units had relatively high casualty rates partly due to being treated like outcasts and sometimes even openly vilified by other unit members. A new accession to a unit as a replacement for a wounded or killed unit member may be particularly ostracized by other unit members until their feelings of grief over the loss of the previous unit member fade. Unit leaders must not allow group dynamics to run their own course as new accessions are incorporated into a unit. Instead, new unit members must be afforded every opportunity to gain necessary skills, prove themselves, and earn the trust of other unit members quickly, safely, and without jeopardizing the unit's cohesion.

> *As casualties grew, replacements did not know the men or leaders with whom they had to fight, they lost confidence because they felt alone and because they were not trained. This had a vicious effect on the cycle of casualties.*
>
> **LtCol R.E. Cushman, USMC**
> *Marine Corps Gazette*

## Keep Unit Members Part of the Unit Even After They Leave

The psychologically protective effects of unit cohesion can evaporate quickly for unit members who transfer out soon after returning or who return ahead of their deployed units because of injury, illness, or a home emergency. Two groups of individuals who are at particular risk for stress reactions or injuries after being abruptly separated from the unit with which they deployed are individual augmentees and members of Selected Reserve units who demobilize immediately upon returning from a war zone deployment.

Likewise, unit members who transfer to other units or who are released from active duty within the first few months of returning from an operational deployment are at increased psychological risk because of their loss of peer support as a resource for resilience and recovery. Unit leaders, especially commanders of combatant units, can minimize this risk by maintaining ongoing contact with all detached or demobilized unit members, even those who leave the Service. E-mail groups that include all current and former members of an operational unit can be useful vehicles for maintaining peer support over long distances. Other resources for maintaining peer support for detached or separated unit members are unit associations that maintain Web sites and blogs and sponsor reunions to help veterans maintain ongoing peer support.

## Ensure Continuity of Leadership

Turnover of key unit leadership during or immediately before or after a deployment can have a devastating effect on unit cohesion, trust, and support. If possible, transfers of leaders at various levels in the unit should be staggered to ensure continuity and to minimize the negative impact of leader turnover. New leaders can limit disruptions in unit cohesion by honoring previous unit leaders and recognizing the respect and admiration unit members may have had for them before making significant changes. Unit leaders who serve with combat units in war zones often consider their leadership roles with members of that unit to be a lifetime job that continues regardless of how far apart unit members drift in subsequent years.

## Zero Tolerance for Hazing or Abuse by Leaders

The more highly stressed individuals become, the more likely they are to experience increased levels of anger and aggressive impulses and decreased ability to control their tempers when frustrated. In addition to outbursts of temper, individuals under stress may also be more likely to display sadistic aggression toward their peers and subordinates in the unit. Hazing and the abuse of subordinates by leaders always damages trust, respect, and teamwork and should never be tolerated.

## Keep Unit Members in Close Contact with Each Other

Regular voice and face-to-face contact between unit members are important to maintaining resilience. Two unit members working or fighting side-by-side are stronger than two unit members working or fighting in separate locations. Examples of situations that erode resilience through interference with direct face-to-face and voice contact include the requirement to wear mission-oriented protective posture gear and the dispersion of unit members across physically separate locations. It is important to be able to recognize individual unit members even while they are wearing mission-oriented protective posture gear, maintain voice contact directly or through radios as much as possible, and keep all periods of visual and auditory isolation from other unit members as brief as possible.

## Mentor Outliers

The cohesion and effectiveness of military units as teams depend on all unit members fitting in, pulling their weight, and earning others' respect and trust. Individuals who lack the experience or capacity to be productive members of a team may become even more corrosive to unit cohesion if they perceive themselves to be openly rejected and publicly criticized. These 5 percent who sometimes require 95 percent of leaders' time and attention must either be mentored fully into the unit by a trusted NCO or petty officer or be separated from the unit and military service.

# Family Support

Almost everyone who deploys with a Marine or Navy unit leaves behind family members or others in the community with whom they have strong bonds and on whom they depend for social support. The degree to which Marines and Sailors depend on family members or other community members as resources for resilience varies greatly and may change quickly due to changes in these sustaining personal relationships. Service members also vary greatly in their tolerance for separation from loved ones and their ability to sustain supportive and constant relationships without physical presence and contact. For many Marines and Sailors, there can be no substitute for ongoing contact and supportive communication with family and community members. Some factors that may contribute to loss of family support include the following:

- Recent marriage or engagement.
- Pregnant wife or new baby.
- No prior experience maintaining a long-distance relationship.

- Significant money or other family problems.
- Spouse lacks support from extended family or the military community.
- Family or relationship breakups.
- Infidelity in a marriage or relationship.
- Family conflicts that can't be resolved during deployment.
- Illnesses or injuries to family members back home.
- Breakdowns or obstacles to family communication.
- Untreated stress reactions, injuries, or illnesses in family members back home.

A blessing or a curse, depending on the nature of the relationship and communication between deployed Marines or Sailors and their significant others, family relationships can either provide valuable resources to augment resilience against in-theater stressors or they can become additional sources of severe stress that saps other resources for resilience. The impact of family relationships on unit member resilience can be very difficult for unit leaders to manage, given how little direct control leaders have over family members and the way they relate to Marines and Sailors in the unit. Leadership efforts in this area can pay large dividends in enhanced health and well-being among unit members and their families. The following paragraphs discuss unit leader actions to enhance and maintain family support as a resilience resource.

## Solve Family Problems Before Deployment Whenever Possible

Problems that seem like molehills while unit members are still at home can quickly become mountains during deployment. While separated, unit members and their spouses and children have few tools at their disposal to solve problems. Families need extensive preventive maintenance before deployments because broken families, unlike pieces of equipment, cannot be swapped out or easily repaired during deployment. Unit Marines and Sailors should be encouraged to inventory their important sources of family and community support long before deployment and anticipate and eliminate any threats to family relationships, health, and well-being whenever possible. Unit leaders with personal experience maintaining strong and supportive family relationships during previous deployments can be invaluable mentors for younger, less experienced unit members.

## Give Unit and Family Members the Skills to Cope Throughout Deployment Cycles

Marines and Sailors spend many months preparing to deploy—learning skills, acquiring knowledge, becoming physically and mentally stronger, and developing teams. Meanwhile, families may become weaker, especially if family members are not trained in the knowledge and skills necessary to function well as a family during deployment. Families need to be trained before, during, and after deployments in the skills they need to thrive through separations and reunions. Numerous resources exist to help unit leaders in the training and support of unit families, including base and station family support organizations, spouse peer support systems, and religious ministry personnel and services. Examples of such organizations include Marine Corps Community Services (MCCS), Navy Fleet and Family Support Center, and the ombudsman and family readiness programs. All of these are resources for the training of family members as they prepare for the Service members' return from deployment; however, none of these resources can be a substitute for the direct leadership of commanders and their chains of command in the important family readiness mission. Though the ultimate responsibility of leaders remains paramount, fielding full-time family readiness officers as extensions of unit leadership for families promises to improve the training and preparation of families for wartime deployments.

## Train Family Members to Recognize Stress Injuries and Illnesses

Every member of a military family, from youngest to oldest, is directly affected by military deployments, especially during times of war. All family members can react to the stress of family separations and other hardships as well as the dangers faced by a spouse or parent deployed to a war zone. Any family member can suffer a stress reaction, injury, or illness due to prolonged or intense stress, such as that caused by losses of friends by death or serious injury, in-theater life-threats experienced vicariously through communication with a deployed Service member or through news media, the wear-and-tear grind of too many responsibilities endured with too little rest, and inner conflicts caused by perceived failures of those in civil or military authority to uphold organizational or cultural values and ethics.

Since a stress injury or illness in any family adds stress to everyone else in the family, early recognition and treatment of these problems, either in the Service member or a family member, is crucial for family resilience. All family members should be given age-appropriate training in the recognition of the four color-coded stress zones of the stress continuum model and in finding the appropriate level of help for each zone.

## Train Unit and Family Members to Communicate Effectively

Communication in families often begins to break down just before deployments. It may suffer prolonged disruption during deployments and afterward due to escalating and irresolvable conflicts. To maintain family support during deployments, unit and family members must develop a communication plan prior to deployment. The plan must include clear guidelines regarding how, when, and what they will communicate during deployment, so that the withholding of information will not be perceived as a withdrawal or an abandonment. After deployments end, family members also need to repair breaches in their communication and trust by listening carefully to each others' experience of the deployment and developing a shared deployment narrative and understanding of the meaning of what they experienced.

## Help Unit and Family Members Solve Family Problems During Deployments

Young Marines, Sailors, and their spouses often have few resources and skills for solving family financial, health, or other problems before deployments and may have even fewer resources for solving such problems later while Service members are deployed. Solving family problems during deployments may be especially challenging for military spouses who are new to the area, have no extended family nearby, and are not comfortable relying on other unit spouses. Unit leaders at all levels should find ways to augment the resources available to families throughout deployment cycles.

# Preserving Spiritual Resources

Although the spiritual dimension of life is one about which opinions and practices greatly vary, it is one that provides many people valuable resources for resilience to stress and recovery from stress injuries whether they realize it or not. To some, spirituality is synonymous with religious practice based on a faith in God. For many, worshipping God as part of a faith community provides a wealth of resources for mastering severe stress. Spirituality, though, has a broader definition that applies even to those individuals who do not believe in God or do not belong to an organized religion. This broader view defines spirituality as an overarching source of meaning that transcends the day-to-day struggles of the individual and helps give life value and meaning. In this broader sense, the Navy and Marine Corps are inherently spiritual organizations and their traditions and core values help Marines, Sailors, and their family members find meaning and value in all that they do. Unit leaders and chaplains can be spiritual teachers to the extent that they mentor their Marines and Sailors to trust in their organization's values and to find meaning in their experiences. Some stressors that can damage meaning and trust in values include the following:

- Witnessing or engaging in ethical violations, especially if condoned by leaders.
- Leaders preaching the unit's core values, but not putting them into practice.
- Failing to adequately honor the fallen.
- Events that don't make sense, logically or morally.
- Leaders failing to acknowledge and correct their own mistakes.
- Uncorrected breaches of discipline.
- Uncorrected breaches of two-way respect.

## Meaning and Trust in Values

All people need to make sense out of their experiences and believe that future events can be predicted based on past experiences and the rules by which the universe appears to work. Imagine how disorienting and frightening it would be to suddenly live in a world where all the old, trusted rules no longer applied—where gravity made objects fall up rather than down, where there were no laws to deter violent crime, and where no one ever spoke one word of truth.

Most people never experience such a challenge to their moral values or other deeply held beliefs; such beliefs operate entirely outside of conscious awareness because life makes sense to them almost all the time. For most, beliefs about the nature of life are permitted to evolve only very slowly over a lifetime as life experience and wisdom accrue.

On the other hand, research on the mental and spiritual components of psychological trauma, loss, and moral injury has shown that one of the defining features of such stress injuries is that they shatter existing assumptions about God, goodness, and the moral order in a way that leaves a void in understanding and meaning. To heal and recover from such injuries requires individuals to reconstruct their core beliefs and trust in values to make new sense out of what has happened and their role in it. Since individuals tend to draw their moral values and core beliefs from the social organizations to which they belong, the leaders of those organizations—including the entire chain of command in a military unit—play a crucial role in conserving trust and meaning in unit members through promoting sturdy and realistic beliefs before deployment and then mentoring unit members to regain trust in values or meaning in life that has been lost during deployment. The following paragraphs discuss leader actions for conserving meaning and trust in values as vital resources for resilience.

## Ethics and Rules Enforcement

Few events can damage trust in moral values more profoundly than actions by leaders or unit members that are perceived to grossly violate professed core values or ethical or legal standards, such as the rules of engagement or the law of war, especially if unit leaders fail to acknowledge and aggressively correct whatever wrongs may have been committed. Such "senseless" events can cause unit members to at least temporarily suspend their own moral codes, seeing them as currently irrelevant and possibly leading to further violations of ethical rules. Ethical misconduct in the unit can also cause lasting damage to individual unit members' internal moral compasses and a loss of trust in their own and others' basic goodness. Moral damage is potentially the greatest when individuals realize, after the excitement and detached numbness of a combat engagement fades, that they have somehow violated their own deeply-held moral code.

Compounding the impact of these failings, communication and trust in a unit that has committed or witnessed ethical violations can be quickly replaced by a conspiracy of silence, accusations, and recriminations. Unit members can feel torn as they are forced to choose between their loyalty to their peers and leaders and their adherence to standards of right and wrong. Leaders' responsibilities to conserve this vital spiritual resource are clear and simple—prevent inner conflict stress injuries by relentlessly enforcing core values and ethical rules and then act swiftly and decisively to restore trust in these values and rules if they have been damaged by unit members' ethical violations. The worst thing a leader can do in such cases is to collude with the conspiracy of silence in the unit by pretending that nothing bad happened. Remember that unit leaders are the guardians of their Service's ethics and values as well as the honor derived from living by them.

## Frequently Reassess Leadership Actions for Consistency with Core Values

Marines and Sailors mimic and become whatever they see in the leaders they admire, regardless of what they are told. All leaders, perhaps even subconsciously, tell their subordinates, "Do as I do, not as I say." Whether leaders like it or not, few of their missteps go unnoticed by subordinates. The honor of the Marine Corps and Navy depends on its members striving to express honor, courage, and commitment in every word and deed. Regular, honest, and humble self-appraisal is essential to becoming an ever-better model of these values.

## Memorial Services, Ceremonies, and Physical Memorials

There is no more profound expression of the core values of the Marine Corps and Navy than when Marines and Sailors voluntarily sacrifice their lives. The honor of heroes past and present must be preserved through memorials and ceremonies of all kinds. Leaders must give meaning to sacrifices and losses in their unit that transcend short-term military objectives and politics.

## After Action Reviews to Restore Meaning and Trust in Values

As described in appendix C, AARs can be valuable tools for unit leaders to listen to their Marines' and Sailors' perceptions of events that may have violated ethical or moral standards and to anticipate their possible mistrust in these values. The goals of AARs in this context are to make clear what really happened; logically and morally make sense out of what happened; and restore lost trust in moral values by correcting misconceptions and honestly addressing actual ethical violations in order to reaffirm fundamental rules, ethics, and core values.

## Ethics Inclusion in All Unit Training and Operations

Marines and Sailors can become more morally resilient by including guided small-group discussions of ethics in all significant training and operations. Every unit action should be explained in terms of organizational core values and ethical standards, such as the rules of engagement and the law of war, and spirituality as a reverence for and dedication to powers greater than the individual.

# Faith in God and Goodness

Not everyone believes in God and those who do believe have widely varied conceptions of the Divine and methods of worship; however, most people want to believe in goodness as a strong, central thread woven through life. A firm belief in goodness is so fundamental to respecting and making sense of life that those who have lost this belief can neither be convinced to go on living, nor be trusted to treat others with basic human compassion and dignity. Unit leaders may have little interest in the nature and depth of their unit members' faith in God or their religious preferences, but leaders have ample reason to monitor and conserve their unit members' beliefs in goodness. The following paragraphs discuss leader actions to conserve faith and goodness as resources for resilience. Some stressors that can damage faith in God and goodness include the following:

- Bad things happening to good people.
- Betrayals of trust by leaders, close peers, or family members.
- Actions about which individuals feel intensely guilty or ashamed (and unforgivable).
- Inability to forgive others.
- Moral dilemmas.

## Be a Model of Compassion, Forgiveness, and Self-Forgiveness

An inability to forgive oneself for personal failings or shortcomings or to forgive others for their transgressions and betrayals is often at the core of chronic, disabling stress illnesses. Losses of faith in God or goodness often coexist with such failures to forgive. Often, the only proof Marines and Sailors can find for the existence of God or goodness in their lives—and the only way they can learn to forgive themselves and others—is through witnessing the consistent modeling of empathy, compassion, and forgiveness in their peers, family members, and leaders.

## Team with the Unit Chaplain to Restore Faith in God

Studies have shown that a strong faith in God can add significantly to resilience, regardless of how that God is understood or worshipped. If unit or family members abandon their faith in God and goodness due to their inability to reconcile war zone experiences with their previous beliefs, unit leaders may team up with unit or base chaplains to address such losses of faith and to try to restore belief systems and religious practices. The restoration of faith, even in an altered and, perhaps, more mature form, can contribute significantly to current psychological health and future resilience. Unit leaders and chaplains, however, must remain mindful that faith is always a uniquely personal experience and that more harm than good can be done by imposing one's own beliefs on someone else.

## Help Unit Members Make Sense Out of Moral Dilemmas

Irresolvable internal conflicts, such as between good and bad or between the way things should be and the way they really are, can quickly erode psychological and spiritual health and well-being. Marines and Sailors may not voluntarily communicate their inner conflicts to chaplains or unit leaders; they may not even be aware of them. A leader or chaplain can promote recovery and resilience by anticipating moral conflicts in the unit and family members. Leaders can help them resolve their dilemmas by listening empathically and resisting the urge to oversimplify or resolve their conflicts.

## Encourage Religious Practice

For those unit members motivated to do so, participating in worship services as part of a faith community and reading sacred texts, such as the Bible, Tanakh, or Koran, can provide valuable spiritual resources for resilience. Unit leaders can make such spiritual resources more readily available to unit members by creating a culture of respect for religious practice and tolerance for religious diversity and by setting aside time in weekly schedules for religious worship.

> *Loss of belief in a loving God, loss of core spiritual values, difficulties reconciling war zone experiences with faith, and a lack of forgiveness have all been correlated with severity of PTSD in combat veterans.*
>
> **Drescher, Smith, and Foy**
> *Combat Stress Injury: Theory, Research, and Management*

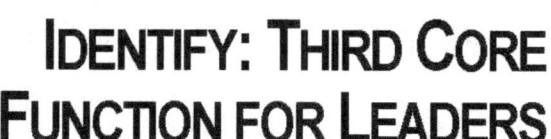

# IDENTIFY: THIRD CORE FUNCTION FOR LEADERS

Individual Marines and Sailors, as perceiving, thinking, and decision-making beings, are the most powerful weapons in the arsenals of the Navy and Marine Corps. Although powerful, Marines and Sailors can never be "fire and forget" weapons. No matter how well-trained and prepared they are, Sailors and Marines need continual *guidance* to make full use of their potentials—keeping their efforts directed toward mission accomplishment—and continual *replenishment* of physical, mental, social, and spiritual resources to remain strong and capable. Leaders must identify—the third core function of leadership in COSC and OSC—the stress zones in which individuals are operating and the stressors by which they are being challenged.

The first three core COSC and OSC functions can be compared with the broad tasks required to operate and maintain a warship in the fleet. In this metaphor, strengthening is like arming and equipping the warship for the specific mission to be accomplished before it gets underway; mitigating is like continually providing the warship with the fuel, ammunition, lubricants, and other resources needed to operate, while keeping the ship well clear of storms, shoals, and other avoidable dangers; and identifying is like closely monitoring every available indicator of ship functioning and performance to quickly recognize when something may have gone wrong and repairs may be needed.

Just as with the operation and maintenance of a ship, the identifying function involves more than looking, listening, and feeling for signs of possible breakage or wear—it suggests anticipating these inevitabilities. Leaders must identify not only the stress reactions, injuries, and illnesses experienced by their Marines and Sailors, but also the day-to-day stressors they encounter so they can recognize occasions of high risk for stress problems. Whereas strengthening and mitigation are activities to promote primary prevention, the core function of identification makes secondary prevention possible—timely interventions that may prevent small problems from becoming big ones.

This chapter reviews the principles and guidelines for the third core COSC and OSC function of identification. It includes how to recognize a Marine's or Sailor's stress zone and which sources of stress may be most likely to push them further to the right—away from health and readiness—on the stress continuum model.

# Identifying Stress Zones

**Unit Leader's Goals for Monitoring Stress Zones:**

Maximize performance

Minimize risk for damage from stress

## The Two Goals of Monitoring Stress Zones

The stress continuum model with its four, color-coded stress zones can be compared to the pressure gauge for a boiler or the tachometer for an engine. It is a visual aid for identifying current operating conditions in the context of the entire possible operating range. It is also a tool used to maximize performance and minimize risk for damage to the mind, brain, or spirit from excessive stress.

## The Stress Continuum Model Dashboard

There are important ways in which the stress continuum model differs from a tachometer or pressure gauge—since human beings never really shut down, even while sleeping, the stress zone of a Marine or Sailor is never zero; and neither engine speed nor boiler pressure can get "pinned" to the far right of their operating ranges indefinitely. Unlike a machine, one of the defining features of the Orange Zone of stress injuries is that once an individual's stress level enters the Orange Zone, it will not immediately return fully to the Green Zone even after sources of stress have been removed.

Although stress injuries are more likely in Marines or Sailors whose stress level has been in the Yellow "Reacting" Zone for a long period of time, stress injuries can also occur to Marines and Sailors who are impacted by a single overwhelming event, such as an unexpected life-threat or the loss of a close peer, even while comfortably in the Green Zone. A unit member's stress level can jump instantly from low (Green) to very high (Orange) without passing through any intermediate levels, something an engine tachometer could never do.

Figure 4-1 depicts how the stress continuum model might look if every Marine and Sailor had a stress instrument panel or "dashboard" like a boiler or engine. Notice that the needle of the "stress-o-meter" to the left of the dashboard is free to swing back and forth between Green and Yellow Zones, since all movements within this narrow range are temporary. Once an Orange Zone stress injury occurs, however, the effects of that injury persist after sources of stress have been removed even though the stress level seems to have returned to the Green Zone. Once a stress injury occurs, the Orange warning light on the stress continuum model dashboard remains lit until the stress injury heals. Healing, discussed more in chapter 5, may take between a few days and a few months.

If Marines and Sailors had a visible stress dashboard, the glowing Orange "Injured" warning light would serve as a signal to leaders, peers, family members, and other injured individuals that there is a problem that requires attention in order to return to full function. The Red "Ill" light would illuminate only if a stress injury did not

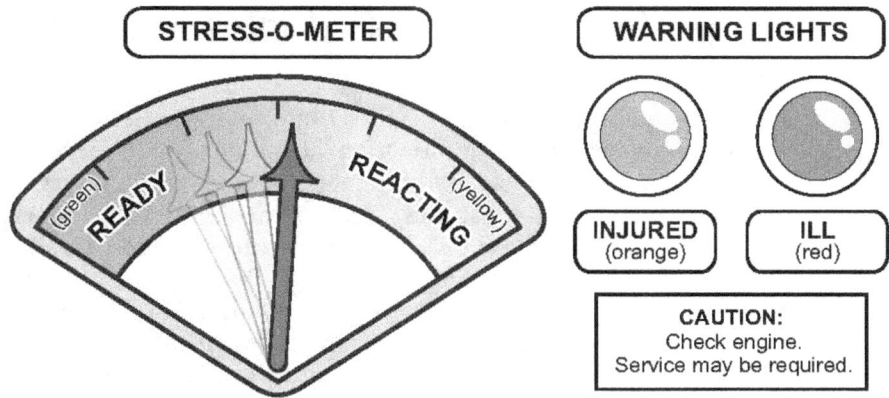

**Figure 4-1.** Combat and Operational Stress Continuum "Dashboard".

heal normally over time, instead producing persistent and worsening symptoms associated with substance abuse or dependence or a mental disorder, such as PTSD, depression, or anxiety. Only a medical or mental health professional can determine whether the red light is lit by diagnosing a stress illness.

## Key Indicators and Sources of Information to Identify Stress Zones

A boiler pressure gauge receives a continuous flow of information about the pressure of gases inside the boiler and an engine tachometer receives continuous information about the rotation of the engine's shaft. What information must unit leaders continuously receive about their Marines and Sailors to keep track of their stress zones and how do they acquire it?

To identify stress zones, leaders must monitor three key indicators of stress (see table 4-1)—the specific stressors from all sources currently or recently experienced by the individual, which contribute to the "stress load" affecting that individual; the level of internal distress, including uncomfortable or troubling thoughts or feelings, such as anxiety, sadness, grief, anger, guilt, or shame; and the effectiveness of functioning in all spheres, including the ability to perform assigned duties, to interact with others appropriately, and to maintain healthy physical functioning. Leaders must answer the following questions to identify the stress zone occupied by their Marines and Sailors:

- What stressors have they recently encountered?
- What is the level of their current internal distress?
- Have their functioning and performance been degraded by stress?

Unit leaders in almost all settings and situations have access to two sources of information about their unit members' recent stressors, levels of internal distress, and effectiveness of functioning—what they see, particularly when observing the behavior of those unit members in various settings, and what they hear, particularly in response to the question, "How are you doing?" Both sources of information—observation and listening—are crucial for unit leaders to accurately assess their unit members' stress zones. Neither can be ignored.

Table 4-1. Indicators and Sources of Stress Zone Information.

| | | Sources of Information | |
|---|---|---|---|
| | | Watch for: | Listen for: |
| Key Indicators | Recent Stressors | Stressors during deployment or training | Personal or home stressors. |
| | Level of Distress | Uncharacteristic and intense negative emotions. | Troubling thoughts, such as guilt or shame. |
| | Level of Functioning | Changes in job performance, self-care, or getting along with others. | Physical symptoms, sleep problems, or loss of self-control. |

# Responsibility for Monitoring Indicators of Stress

As with the other core functions of COSC and OSC, unit commanders always retain primary responsibility for identifying stress zones in unit members and their families; however, commanding officers cannot perform this task without help or input from others. Commanding officers receive information to help identify stress zones not only from individual Marines and Sailors, but also from family members, peers, members of the chain of command, and unit medical and religious ministry personnel. To accurately identify unit members' stress zones, commanders must consider all available information (see fig 4-2).

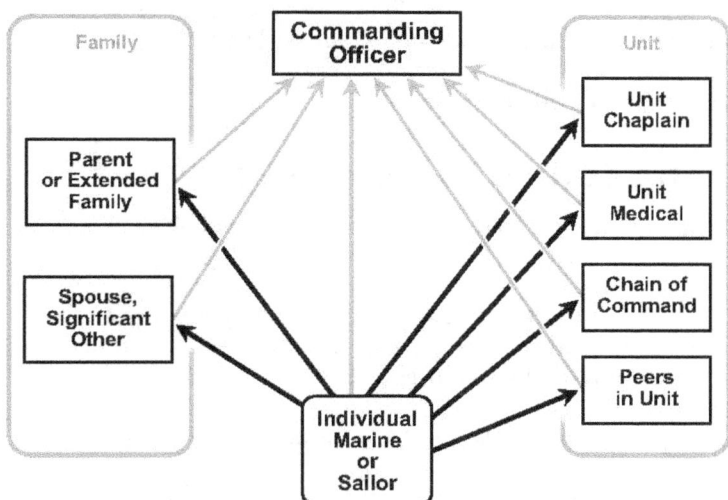

Figure 4-2. Flow of Stress Indicator.

# Recognizing the Green "Ready" Zone

The Green "Ready" Zone is the stress state of individuals who are physically and psychologically healthy and functioning up to their full capacities, despite the stressors they face. The Green Zone is defined by the absence of significant distress or losses of functioning, but it also encompasses positive states of wellness and enhanced performance, such as those resulting from the mastery of challenges; creative problem solving; and physical, social, and spiritual fitness. The Green Zone is the goal toward which all COSC and OSC and psychological health efforts are directed—before, during, and after deployments. Though the Green Zone is the goal, leaders must understand that the intensity and duration of modern war zone stressors and the training to prepare for them can push their Marines and Sailors out of this zone again and again. In arduous deployments to war zones, Marines and Sailors may rarely function in the Green Zone, although they continually strive to return to it.

## Green Zone Stressors

The stressors experienced by Marines and Sailors operating in the Green Zone may be of any type, magnitude, or duration. The defining feature of the Green Zone is not a particular set of outcomes caused by a particular set of stressors; rather, it is continued well-being and optimal performance in spite of them. The greater the intensity and duration of stressors, the more likely they are to push Marines and Sailors out of the Green Zone. Every individual has unique capacities and vulnerabilities that change over time based on current stress load, duration of stressor exposure, and available resources.

## Green Zone Characteristics

Green Zone characteristics (see table 4-2) may be evident in the following attributes:

- In full control of body and mind, including emotions.
- Focused on mission performance, as required.
- Calm and poised under pressure.
- Self-confident.
- Able to solve complex problems rationally and creatively.
- Quick to recover from fear or anger.
- Not preoccupied with blame of self or anyone else.
- Has a sense of humor.
- Focused on important issues and doesn't worry needlessly.

- Flexible in adapting to new or changing situations.
- Relaxed and sleeps soundly when time is available.
- Enjoys play and other social activities with peers when not working.
- Listens empathically to others and thinks about others' welfare.
- Places mission and others' welfare above own.
- Morally and phsically courageous.

Table 4-2. Examples of Green "Ready" Zone Indicators.

| Current Stressors | No or few casualties in unit. | "Everything's OK with my family at home." |
|---|---|---|
| | Unit members are well and prepared for deployment. | "Deploying isn't so tough." |
| | Unit is accomplishing mission. | "Give me something else to do, I'm bored." |
| | Unit members are busy, but get adequate rest. | |
| Level of Distress | Smooth teamwork. | "I'm good to go." |
| | Consistent mission focus. | "I'll do it." |
| | Humor and play, when possible. | "I can fix this problem." |
| | No fighting or hazing. | "I'm not worried." |
| Changes in Functioning | Able to sleep soundly. | "I'm getting enough sleep." |
| | Good control of emotions. | "I am confident." |
| | Self-confidence. | "I am healthy and fit." |
| | Concern for others. | "My Marines and Sailors are doing well." |
| | Moral and physical courage. | |

# Recognizing the Yellow "Reacting" Zone

The Yellow "Reacting" Zone is the state in which individuals operate when they have experienced mild and temporary distress or loss of normal functioning because of stress. Central to the definition of Yellow Zone stress reactions is that they are never severe or long-lasting. Yellow Zone distress and losses of function always go away soon after the source of stress has been removed or neutralized. They often improve significantly as soon as the individual has mastered a new challenge and adapted to it.

Yellow Zone stress reactions are not necessarily negative experiences to be avoided at all costs. Without Yellow Zone stress intentionally induced during tough training and operational experience, Marines and Sailors would never develop the strength, endurance, self-confidence, and skill needed to perform their duties under arduous conditions. All training, if it is of the optimal intensity, intentionally induces Yellow Zone reactions. In the same way that stress on the muscular system, intentionally applied during physical training, is essential for the development of muscle mass and strength, stress on the mind, brain, and spirit are essential for the development of psychological strength. The potential problems with Yellow Zone stress reactions—and the reasons they should be closely monitored by leaders—is the risk such reactions bring for suboptimal mental performance while under intense stress and for possible Orange Zone stress injuries if Yellow Zone stress persists. Training so hard for a military mission that unit members incur Orange Zone stress injuries is as counterproductive as training so hard for a sporting event, such as a marathon race, that one limps up to the starting line on race day.

Understanding the usual course of Yellow Zone stress reactions is helpful for anticipating and recognizing them (see fig. 4-3). Yellow Zone reactions are most likely to occur at the beginning and ending of each new challenge or any time new challenges are heaped on top of existing ones. If a new challenge lasts long enough for Marines and Sailors to successfully master it, most get into a "groove" of Green Zone adaptation at some point between the onset and end of the stressor. Those who do not achieve Green Zone adaptation may be hampered by individual resources, preparation, or any other stressor experienced at the same moment, including those in their personal and family lives.

## Yellow Zone Stressors

The stressors that usually cause Yellow Zone stress reactions are generally *not* those associated with a life-threat or other intense

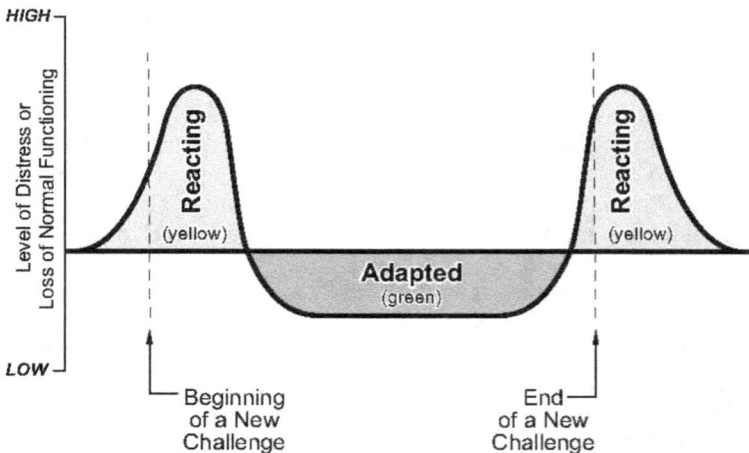

Figure 4-3. Usual Course of Yellow Zone Stress Reactions.

and potentially overwhelming experiences in a combat zone. Rather, Yellow Zone stressors tend to be the commonplace annoyances, irritations, conflicts, worries, and other challenges that everyone experiences every day. Since Yellow Zone stressors are extremely common (see table 4-3), so also are Yellow Zone stress reactions. Everyone experiences stress reactions in the Yellow Zone and some people spend most of their time reacting to stress from one source or another. The factors that determine whether those individuals will experience mild and transient distress or functional impairment, such as a stress reaction, at any given moment are the stressors impinging on that individual at that point in time and the resources currently available to him for coping and mastering stress. The important characteristics of Yellow Zone stressors are—

- Commonplace, occurring every day.
- Only mild to moderate in severity.
- Come from many different sources, including the physical, mental, social, and spiritual dimensions.
- Come from within and outside the unit, such as operational or personal/home sources.
- No stressor is intense enough to be overwhelming by itself.
- Additive over time, Yellow Zone stressors may pile up on each other like the proverbial straws that threaten to break the camel's back.

**Table 4-3.** Examples of Common Sources of Yellow Zone Stress.

|  | Physical | Mental | Social | Spiritual |
|---|---|---|---|---|
| **Operational Sources** | Harsh weather. Rough terrain. Cramped, uncomfortable spaces. Minor injuries. Sleep deprivation. Poor nutrition. Lack of opportunities for exercise. | Ambiguous or difficult missions. Uncertainty. Lack of information. Unfamiliarity with mission or environment. Boredom. Prolonged concentration. | Being surrounded by strangers, as is the case with individual augmentees. Conflicts with peers or leaders. Lack of personal space. Working in isolation. Hostility from foreign nationals. | Inner conflicts over competing values. Difficulty making sense of what happens. Strain on commitment to organization. Disillusionment regarding mission. |
| **Personal Sources** | Money problems. Loss of personal possessions. Minor illnesses. Alcohol misuse or abuse. | Worries about welfare of family. Helplessness to deal with family problems. Uncertainties about the future. | Conflicts with spouse or family. Relationship breakups. Loss of contact with family. Missing friends. | Strain on belief in God. Divided loyalties between military and family. Loss of ability to practice faith. |

# Yellow Zone Signs of Distress or Changes in Functioning

Although inwardly directed negative emotions, such as anxiety, sadness, worry, and fear, also occur, distress in the Yellow Zone often takes the form of outwardly directed negative emotions, such as irritation, frustration, and anger (see table 4-4). Marines and Sailors who experience any of these uncharacteristic negative emotions while in the Yellow Zone may be completely unaware of their own internal distress, especially in operational environments that require them to be tough, stoic, and outwardly focused. Other unit members may be more aware of an individual's internal distress because of the uncharacteristic behaviors they witness that externally reflect such internal distress. These include angry outbursts, worrying out loud, or withdrawal from normal social interactions. Even Marines and Sailors who seem oblivious to their own internal distress will usually give a truthful and insightful answer to the question, "How are you doing?" if it is asked in a way that communicates genuine interest and concern. Some Marines and Sailors operating in the Yellow Zone may not stop to think about how they are feeling and functioning until being asked by someone they trust.

Changes in functioning in the Yellow Zone are likewise mild and transient, although they can affect any aspect of performance including physical, mental, social, and spiritual functioning. Since Yellow Zone stress reactions are diverse and can include any change in functioning, leaders and concerned peers must know and monitor their Marines and Sailors closely enough to recognize every change in behavior. Examples of Yellow Zone changes in functioning are—

- Difficulty relaxing or falling asleep.
- Muscle tension or headaches.
- Changes in appetite (eating too much or too little).
- Weight gain or weight loss.
- Changes in bowel function (diarrhea or constipation).
- Talking too fast or too slowly.
- Becoming uncharacteristically quiet.
- Loss of normal energy, enthusiasm, or interest in life.
- Ceasing or avoiding physical fitness training.
- Difficulty focusing on tasks at hand.

- Difficulty remembering or performing calculations.
- Difficulties following complex instructions.
- Difficulty staying calm and controlling anger or fear.
- Apathy or complacency.
- Not enjoying usual social or recreational activities.
- Withdrawing from normal social interactions.
- Questioning previous beliefs about mission and purpose.

Table 4-4. Examples of Yellow "Reacting" Zone Indicators.

| To Identify: | Watch for: | Listen for: |
|---|---|---|
| **Current Stressors** | Tough mission. High operating tempo. Little time off for rest. Sleep deprivation. Unit mission unclear or changing. Hardships. Real dangers. Few casualties or accidental injuries in unit. | "My wife isn't handling this deployment well." "My girlfriend isn't answering my e-mails." "I am worried about my sick child." "My wife has to take a second job to pay bills." "Some of the guys in the unit hate me." |
| **Level of Distress** | Decreased efficiency of teamwork. Less humor or play. Increased conflicts in unit. Fighting or cruel teasing. Outbursts of temper. Unit members avoiding each other. Dead quiet in berthing areas. | "Everything is pissing me off these days." "I can't stop worrying." "What's the use? This is all a waste of time." "Can I get transferred to another unit?" "I need to get home to my family." |
| **Changes in Functioning** | Loss of focus on the mission. Cutting corners in work. Decreased pride in work. Difficulty getting to sleep. Increased use of sick bay or unit medical. Weight gain or weight loss. Difficulty making sound decisions. Loss of energy and enthusiasm. | "I am not sleeping very well." "There's something wrong with me. I must be sick." "My head feels foggy all the time." "I keep forgetting things." "I keep losing my temper and saying mean things, even though I try not to." "I don't think I can do my job any longer." |

# Recognizing the Orange "Injured" Zone

In stark contrast to the Yellow Zone, the Orange "Injured" Zone is characterized by moderate to severe distress or changes in functioning that persist to some extent even after sources of stress are removed. While Yellow Zone stress reactions are truly normal reactions to stressful events, Orange Zone stress injuries, like any other injury to a person, are not "normal." These reactions indicate that something has been damaged in the person and normal functioning has been degraded. The nature of Orange Zone stress injuries and their distinction from Yellow Zone stress reactions point directly to the reasons why it is so crucial for unit leaders at all levels to accurately recognize Orange Zone injuries as soon as they occur, so they can be appropriately managed and treated (see table 4-5).

Table 4-5. Comparison of Yellow and Orange Zone Stress.

| Yellow Zone Stress Reactions | Orange Zone Stress Injuries |
|---|---|
| Bending under stress. | Partly damaged by stress. |
| Involves whole person: body, mind, and spirit. | Involves whole person: body, mind, and spirit. |
| Partly determined by individual coping choices. | Outside individual control— "snapped" or "lost it." |
| Individual still feels like normal self. | Individual doesn't feel like normal self. |
| Always goes away completely. | Usually heals, but may leave a mental scar. |
| If lasts too long, can lead to an Orange Zone injury. | If doesn't heal, can lead to a Red Zone stress illness. |
| Helped by mitigation. | Helped by treatment. |

The idea that stress can inflict literal injuries to the mind, brain, and spirit is a recent advancement in stress science. The word "trauma" literally means "wound" in its original Greek, but, when applied to stress illnesses, such as PTSD, this word has historically been taken figuratively rather than literally. There is now compelling evidence from studies of stress in humans and animals that the wounds created by overwhelming stress are not merely metaphorical, but as literal as the wounds created in the rest of the body by projectiles, fire, or other impacts.

This crucial distinction has many significant consequences. For example, imagine how differently Marines and Sailors would be treated by unit leaders and medical caregivers who believed that no amount of physical exertion, activity, or impact could result in a literal injury to muscles, bones, and joints. Instead of being examined and treated for possible fractures, sprains, and strains, anyone who developed pain or loss of normal functioning in a limb might simply be told to "suck it up" and get back to duty, regardless of how badly they hurt. Small problems might worsen to become bigger problems through being ignored and anyone who could no longer function in the military because of limb pain or abnormal functioning might be administratively discharged as unsuitable rather than being awarded medical discharges.

This hypothetical scenario may seem ridiculous because the evidence for literal damage to bones, joints, and muscles from wear and tear or intense impacts is overwhelming and undeniable. Even without the benefit of an x-ray, most people can recognize severe fractures or sprains just from how they appear. Since stress injuries are far less visible to the naked eye and there are not yet any foolproof diagnostic tests for them, the prevailing view since World War I has been that stress problems arising in combat or other military operations are due to personal weakness or a lack of motivation over literal physical or mental damage.

In light of modern science, this view no longer makes sense. Furthermore, since the Marine Corps and Navy have begun acknowledging that stress of sufficient intensity or duration can inflict injuries to the brain, mind, and spirit of a Marine or Sailor, the social stigma associated with admitting to having significant stress problems has been reduced in the Department of the Navy and individuals needing care to recover more quickly and completely from stress injuries have been more willing to seek it.

Compared with Yellow Zone stress reactions, the distress and changes in function associated with Orange Zone stress injuries tend to have a more abrupt onset and to persist significantly longer, well beyond the disappearance of the stressor that inflicted the stress injury (see fig. 4-4 on page 4-14). The intensity of Orange Zone stress injury symptoms also tends to change more quickly over time, especially in the first few seconds or minutes after the moment of stress injury. This phenomenon is similar to the pain experienced after a significant physical injury, such as a serious burn or the fracture of a bone. Individuals who sustain such physical injuries usually experience the immediate onset of very intense discomfort that partially fades over the next few minutes, although discomfort and changes in function will persist to a varying extent for quite a while longer, perhaps weeks, months, or even years. Also like physical injuries, the usual, expected course for Orange Zone stress injuries is to heal over time unless something prevents healing.

## Orange Zone Stressors

Orange Zone stressors, much less common than Yellow Zone stressors, can occur in any operational environment—on land, sea, or air and in peacetime or war. Unlike Yellow Zone stress reactions, which can be caused by many physical, mental, social, and spiritual challenges, Orange Zone stress injuries are typically caused by only four different types of stressors (see table 4-6)—

- Life-threat.
- Loss.
- Inner conflict.
- Wear and tear.

The first three of these four causes of Orange Zone stress injuries are usually single, discrete events. In the case of life-threat, the causative event is usually an unexpected and close brush with death, either nearly being killed or witnessing the death of someone else with whom one identifies or feels close. A close brush with death by itself is not enough to cause a life-threat stress injury as evidenced by the great number of individuals who experience close brushes with death every day without suffering intense and persistent distress or alterations in functioning. In order to produce a stress injury, a life-threatening experience must be of sufficient intensity for that person at that moment to cause literal

> Identifying Orange Zone stress injuries is a crucial reponsibility of unit leaders because Marines and Sailors operating in the Orange Zone are at elevated risk for impairment of both occupational performance and long-term psychological health.

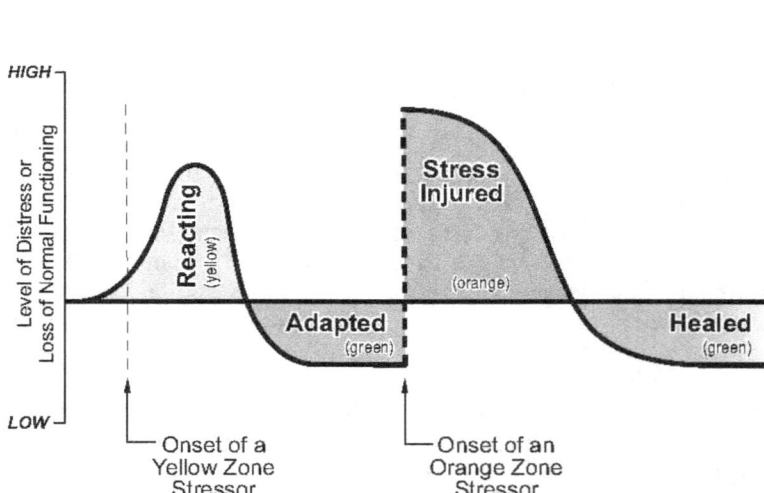

**Figure 4-4.** Comparison of Yellow and Orange Zone Stress.

damage to the nervous system or core beliefs of that individual. The person experiences damage to the brain or mind from a life-threat stress injury as an abrupt loss of control over thinking, feeling, and behaving and it is accompanied by intense feelings of terror, horror, or helplessness. These feelings are never normal for a Marine or Sailor, nor are these feelings of loss of emotional control normal for the spouses and children of Service members. If they occur, they are indicators of possible stress injury.

The second of the four causes of an Orange Zone stress injury is the loss of someone or something that is held dear to the individual. Such a loss could be a death or serious injury of someone, such as a spouse, friend, shipmate, battle buddy, or other member of one's unit. Significant loss injuries can also be caused by relationship breakups, the destruction or other loss of important personal possessions as commonly happens in natural disasters, and the loss of physical integrity and health, such as from an amputation or the loss of other physical functions.

Table 4-6. Examples of Orange Zone Stressors.

|  | In the Field | Underway | In the Home |
|---|---|---|---|
| **Life-Threat** | Being seriously injured in combat. Nearly being killed. Seeing someone else die up close. Handling bodies or body parts. Multiple casualty events, such as IED blasts or ambushes. | Being seriously injured in an accident. Nearly being killed in an accident. Seeing someone else die up close. Handling bodies or body parts. | Being seriously injured in an accident or disaster. Nearly being killed in an accident/disaster. Seeing someone else die up close. Being physically or sexually assaulted. |
| **Loss** | Death of a close friend. Death of a unit member or leader. Loss of valued possessions. | Death of a close friend. Death of a shipmate or leader. Loss of valued possessions. | Relationship breakup. Death or serious injury of a spouse or child. Death of a close friend. |
| **Inner Conflict** | Leaders failing to live up to core values. Failing to save the life of a unit member. Killing or witnessing the killing of a woman or child. Violations of rules of engagement. Friendly fire. | Leaders failing to live up to core values. Failing to save the life of a shipmate. Seeing foreign nationals living in squalor. Inflicting or witnessing violent abuse on a shipmate. | Betrayal of trust by spouse or significant other. Failing to prevent the injury or death of a family member. |
| **Wear and Tear** | Too much Yellow Zone stress for too long. | Too much Yellow Zone stress for too long. | Too much Yellow Zone stress for too long. |

Just as with life-threat stress injuries, individual Marines and Sailors and their family members differ significantly in their vulnerability to suffering severe distress or changes in functioning due to the loss of someone or something important. Individuals also differ regarding the time course of stress injury symptoms due to loss—some experience intense distress and alterations in functioning immediately after a loss, while others suffer such symptoms only later, such as after returning from a combat deployment or underway period. Most people who lose someone they care about deeply experience some degree of Orange Zone stress injury symptoms.

The third event that can cause Orange Zone stress injuries—inner conflict—is the one about which medical and psychological scientists know the least, even though it has been part of human experience for as long as humans have existed. Inner conflict has also been called "moral injury," "betrayal of what's right," or "shattered assumptions" and is caused by events that violate deeply held beliefs, especially codes of conduct and moral codes regarding right and wrong. Inner conflict stress injuries can result when individuals either act or fail to act in ways that violate their own deeply held beliefs and moral codes. It can also occur when trusted others—especially spouses, close friends, or trusted leaders—either act or fail to act in ways that violate these same core beliefs and moral codes. The distress and changes in functioning that can result from an inner conflict stress injury can be just as profound and long-lasting as those resulting from a life-threat or loss.

The fourth Orange Zone stressor is not a single event; rather, it is the accumulation of stress from multiple sources over a long period of time. Wear and tear is caused by the persistence of Yellow Zone stress for too long without sufficient resources for recovery, especially sleep and rest. Unlike the other three types of Orange Zone stress injuries, wear-and-tear stress is more gradual in onset and slower to improve. Wear-and-tear stress injuries are biological in origin. They seem to be caused by the depletion of necessary messenger chemicals in the brain followed by other changes that are the brain's attempt to cope with such chemical depletion. Wear-and-tear stress injuries can be very slow to heal without medical intervention and treatment and can easily lead to lifelong problems. For that reason, it is crucial for leaders of Marines and Sailors to prevent wear-and-tear stress injuries by ensuring adequate sleep, rest, and recovery opportunities for those suffering from Yellow Zone stress. Fortunately, wear and tear is the most preventable of all Orange Zone stressors.

## Orange Zone Signs of Distress or Changes in Functioning

The defining feature of an Orange Zone stress injury is the appearance of moderate to severe distress or alterations in functioning that are outside a person's normal range of experience and beyond his ability to fully control. One of the key features is at least a transient loss of control of aspects of one's body, thoughts, or emotions, occurring either at the time of the Orange Zone stressor event or developing later in response to reminders of that event. Some of these Orange Zone losses of control are observable by others, such as leaders, peers, or family members, while others may be only apparent to the stress-injured individual. Table 4-7, on page 4-18, lists examples of Orange Zone losses of control that can occur until the stress injury heals. These Orange Zone symptoms may be experienced by a stress-injured individual regardless of whether that injury was caused by events involving life-threat, loss, or inner conflict, or merely the wear and tear of smaller stressors accumulating over time.

Appendix F, *Orange Zone Behavior Warning Signs*, describes changes in behavior that may be observed at the time of a life-threat stress injury. None of these changes in behavior proves that an Orange Zone stress injury has definitely occurred, but all should be considered warning signs to prompt further information gathering to identify the stress zone (see table 4-8 on page 4-19). In research with Marine veterans of the wars in Iraq and Afghanistan, all of these behaviors have been found to correlate with later PTSD. Each of the 15 specific behaviors on the checklist should be considered present only if it represents a change from normal baseline behavior for that individual. Because stress injuries are not always evident as observable changes in behavior, appendix F cannot be a substitute for talking with and listening to the individual, especially by asking, "How are you doing?"

**Table 4-7.** Examples of Orange Zone Losses of Control.

|  | **Watch for:** |
|---|---|
| **Body** | Heart pounding hard, even at rest.<br>Shaking, even when not in danger.<br>Sweating, even at rest and when not feeling hot.<br>Loss of control of bladder or bowels.<br>Part of one's body going numb.<br>Being unable to move part of one's body.<br>Transient loss of vision or hearing. |
| **Thinking** | Loss of ability to recall memories.<br>Memories that keep intruding on thinking, even when trying not to remember them.<br>Memories that are so vivid they seem like they are happening now rather than in the past.<br>Painful thoughts or images that keep popping into awareness and can't easily be pushed aside.<br>Violent images or thoughts that keep popping into awareness and can't easily be pushed aside.<br>Loss of ability to mentally concentrate and focus.<br>Losing track of time and surroundings. |
| **Feeling** | Intense and uncharacteristic anger.<br>Sudden outbursts of rage.<br>Intense and uncharacteristic fear.<br>Sudden attacks of panic.<br>Recurring, painful feelings of guilt or shame.<br>Intense and persistent sadness. |

Table 4-8. Examples of Orange "Injured" Zone Indicators.

| To Identify: | Watch for: | Listen for: |
|---|---|---|
| **Current Stressors** | Close brush with death during operational deployment or training. | "I almost got killed in a motorcycle crash yesterday." |
| | The loss of friends, peers, or leaders by death or serious injury. | "My son is very sick and may not pull through." |
| | Events in which actions or failures to act may violate deeply held beliefs or moral values. | "My mom just died." |
| | | "I can't believe my wife cheated on me while we were deployed." |
| | Yellow Zone stress reactions that continue, day after day, for many months. | "My wife left me, taking the kids and all our stuff." |
| **Level of Distress** | Pacing or persistent agitation. | "I can't stop seeing the same scene replayed over and over again in my mind." |
| | Uncharacteristic outbursts of anger, anxiety, or fear. | |
| | Uncharacteristic fighting, alcohol abuse, or misconduct. | "I keep waking up from the same nighmare." |
| | Persistent sadness or absence of normal emotions. | "I don't have any energy anymore." |
| | | "It was all my fault." |
| | Loss of interest in work, hobbies, or socializing. | "I don't trust anyone in this unit any longer." |
| | Persistent withdrawal from interactions with others. | |
| **Changes in Functioning** | Significant and persistent changes in personality. | "I can't slow down my heart rate." |
| | | "I haven't slept in weeks." |
| | Uncharacteristic poor hygiene or grooming. | My appetite is gone, and I have lost a lot of weight." |
| | Sudden drop in job performance. | |
| | Persistent forgetfulness. | "I am afraid I might lose it and hurt someone." |
| | Uncharacteristic emotional loss of control. | |

# Recognizing the Red "Ill" Zone

Most Orange Zone stress injuries heal within days, weeks, or months. The reasons why certain stress injuries don't heal in certain individuals at certain points in time are not yet understood by medical or psychological science. Regardless of the reasons, when an Orange Zone stress injury fails to heal or seems to progressively worsen over time, the individual enters the Red "Ill" Zone. Marines, Sailors, and family members in the Red Zone have stress illnesses that can only be diagnosed by a trained and licensed medical or mental health professional. All Red Zone stress illnesses need professional medical or mental health treatment; however, not all stress illnesses will result in a medical disability discharge from active duty. In fact, only a small percentage of Marines and Sailors who are diagnosed and treated for stress illnesses, such as PTSD, depression, or anxiety, receive a medical discharge. With proper treatment, most will recover and continue their careers and lives either within or outside the military.

Medical science has debated over many centuries about how to distinguish between an injury and an illness or disease. The clearest distinction made between injury and illness may be the oldest—that credited to the ancient Greek physician and the father of modern medicine, Hippocrates. Sometime around the year 400 BC, Hippocrates said that an illness or disease is made up of two components, both of which are necessary for an illness to exist (see *Relations Between Mechanisms of CNS Arousal and Mechanisms of Stress*).

The first component is a wound, injury, or other disruption in the body. The Greek word Hippocrates used for this first component of illness was *pathos*, which literally meant "that which happens to a person to cause suffering." The second component of illness, according to Hippocrates, was embodied in the Greek word *ponos*, which means "toil" or "work." According to Hippocrates, an illness occurs when the body works to heal an injury or other disruption in normal functioning in a way that not only doesn't lead to immediately healing, but also causes other symptoms and problems added on top of the original wound.

A good example is an infection, which is an illness caused by the invasion of the body by bacteria or other microorganisms (the *pathos*), followed by inflammation and other active responses by the body in its effort to fight off the invasion (the *ponos*), which leads to swelling, pain, and other symptoms. In this simple, ancient, relevant view, the difference between an Orange Zone stress injury and a Red Zone stress illness is that a stress illness is a stress injury that the body and mind have unsuccessfully attempted to heal, such that distress and changes in functioning may have become worse instead of better. This ancient definition of illness points the way for modern medical and mental health professionals who work to prevent and treat stress illnesses. Stress illnesses heal when the obstacles to healing are found and eliminated so the mind's natural healing processes work appropriately.

Military leaders should learn to identify Red Zone stress illnesses. Though unit commanders cannot diagnose stress illnesses, they are responsible for closely monitoring their Marines, Sailors, and family members for signs of possible Red Zone stress illness for the following reasons:

- Along with family members, unit leaders are in the best position to recognize the signs that a stress illness may exist in order to ensure early diagnosis and treatment.
- Only unit leaders can ensure that Marines or Sailors with stress illnesses receive a proper and complete course of treatment.
- Sailors and Marines recovering from Red Zone stress illnesses depend on their leaders to help them reintegrate with their units and regain the trust of their peers after treatment has been successful.
- Military leaders have a unique capacity to reduce the stigma associated with recognition and treatment for a stress illness.

## Common Types of Red Zone Stress Illnesses

Table 4-9, on page 4-20, lists the most common Red Zone stress illnesses that may result from unhealed stress injuries caused by each of the four main types of Orange Zone stressors. Many specific stress illnesses may arise from several different types of unhealed stress illness. Furthermore, it is common for several different stress illnesses to occur at the same time in the same individual. Common to all stress illnesses is a high likelihood of abuse or dependence on substances, such as alcohol or drugs, and an increased risk for aggression and other forms of misconduct.

# Red Zone Signs of Distress or Changes in Functioning

Since Red Zone stress illnesses are unhealed and often worsening stress injuries, the signs of distress or alterations in functioning that characterize them are largely the same as those listed in table 4-8 for the Orange "Injured" Zone. The major indicator of a possible stress illness in the Red Zone is the persistence and worsening of stress injury symptoms for many weeks or months after the source of stress injury has been removed, such as after returning from deployment.

Appendix G, *Stress Continuum Decision Flowchart for Marines and Sailors*, is designed to guide leaders to identify stress zones in their Marines and Sailors. The indicators of stress zone listed in the flowchart are a condensed form of those described for each of the four stress zones discussed in this chapter. Appendix H, *Stress Continuum Decision Flowchart for Spouses*, and appendix I, *Stress Continuum Decision Flowchart for Children*, are designed to help identify the current stress zones of family members.

**Table 4-9.** Red Zone Stress Illnesses Arising from Each Orange Zone Stressor Type.

| Life-Threat | Loss | Inner Conflict | Wear and Tear |
|---|---|---|---|
| Acute stress disorder. PTSD. Panic disorder. Alcohol abuse or dependence. Drug abuse or dependence. | Prolonged grief disorder. Major depression. Alcohol abuse or dependence. Drug abuse or dependence. | Disorders of impulse control (especially aggression). Major depression. Generalized anxiety disorder. Alcohol abuse or dependence. Drug abuse or dependence. | Major depression. Generalized anxiety disorder. Alcohol abuse or dependence. Drug abuse or dependence. |

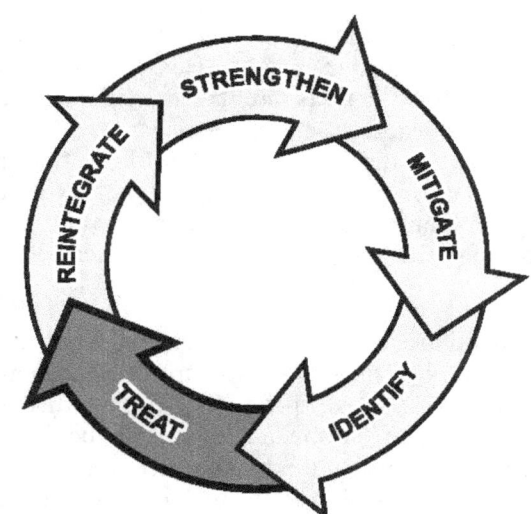

# TREAT: FOURTH CORE FUNCTION FOR LEADERS

In the past, some leaders believed they had little responsibility for the treatment of significant psychological problems experienced by their unit and family members. Treatment, they reasoned, was the responsibility of unit medical personnel and chaplains, backed up by psychologists and psychiatrists in the hospitals. It was not the domain of commanding officers, senior enlisted leaders, or their chains of command; moreover, according to this reasoning, any Marine or Sailor who needed such treatment probably needed to be removed from the unit and replaced with someone who could be better relied upon to do the job under all conditions.

Certain aspects of this argument continue to make sense. For example, it is still true that the diagnosis and professional treatment of Red Zone stress illnesses is largely the direct responsibility of licensed medical and mental health professionals; however, the early and effective treatment of Orange Zone stress injuries and Yellow Zone stress reactions is impossible without the direct leadership of unit commanders and the active participation of their chains of command, families, and individual Service members. Even for Red Zone stress illnesses, unit commanders and their subordinate leaders retain a great responsibility to ensure a full and adequate course of treatment, to monitor progress toward recovery, and to mentor Service members either back to full duty or into a new life as a veteran Marine or Sailor.

For the purposes of COSC and OSC, "intervention" should be broadly defined as all actions taken to promote healing and hasten recovery from stress reactions, injuries, and illnesses, regardless of where or by whom those actions are taken. This chapter describes a set of tools that leaders, Service members, and family members, can employ across the zones of the stress continuum model and across the span of time from the point of maximum stress to the point of maximum recovery. These tools work with the leadership actions for the mitigation of stress described in chapter 3.

Before describing in detail the many treatment actions leaders can take to promote the recovery of their Sailors, Marines, and family members from severe stress, it is worthwhile to first discuss another crucial responsibility commanders and subordinate leaders have with respect to stress and mental health treatment—fighting and defeating the social stigma attached to mental health problems. Stigma is the greatest obstacle to psychological health in the military and, as a barrier to treatment at any level, is costly. Stigma decreases organizational efficiency, damages families, and increases the risk for chronic mental disorders and personal suffering. Stigma makes problems much harder to fix once they are finally treated.

# Stigma: The Greatest Obstacle to Psychological Health in the Military

The word "stigma" literally means "brand" or "mark." When used to describe the way individuals who suffer from mental health problems are perceived by others, the term "social stigma" refers to an invisible mark that sets them apart from their peers and makes them a target for possible ridicule or harm.

Because individuals labeled as having mental health problems are immersed in the same culture as those who might think less of them for it, they often share the same negative attitudes toward their own mental health problems. Hence, those with mental health problems may feel intense shame in addition to being treated differently by the people around them. Social stigma is not unique to the military, nor is it unique to social attitudes about mental health problems; however, mental health stigma can be a serious obstacle to military missions of all kinds and it is inconsistent with the core values of the Navy and Marine Corps.

Stigma is a form of discrimination based on prejudice and stereotyping. It is fueled by ignorance and leaves injustice in its wake. Fighting and defeating stigma is the job of everyone in the military, especially military leaders, who have the greatest influence over the attitudes of Marines, Sailors, and their families.

Mental health stigma, both in and out of the military, takes many forms (see table 5-1). Organizational stigma is based in policies, procedures, and informal rules about worthiness to contribute to the mission. Peer stigma is derived from the language and behaviors that groups use to include or exclude members. Self stigma occurs when individuals suffering from stress problems unfairly blame themselves for those challenges after having absorbed negative attitudes about stress from those around them. All these forms of stigma are based in ignorance and can be defeated with knowledge, awareness, and understanding. Teaching these important stigma-defeating qualities is the responsibility of Navy and Marine Corps leaders.

> *Mental health stigma—based on stereotyping, prejudice, and discrimination—limits career opportunities and discourages those suffering from mental health problems from seeking or accepting help.*
>
> **Patrick Corrigan**
> *American Psychologist*

**Table 5-1.** Sources of Stigma and How to Attack Them.

| Source of Stigma | How to Attack the Source of Stigma |
|---|---|
| Real harm to a military career or future employability specifically because of a mental health diagnosis and treatment. | Ensure that career opportunities are based solely on capabilities and performance, not mental health labels or prejudice. |
| Warrior cultures that place a great value on strength, but may be intolerant of weakness of any kind, whether physical, mental, or moral. | Continuously promote awareness that a wound, injury, or illness—however incurred—is not a sign of weakness. Rather, seeking needed help for any problem is a sign of strength. |
| The belief that stress or mental health problems only happen to individuals who are mentally or morally weak. | Admit openly to your own stress problems in the past and encourage subordinate leaders to do the same. Teach the truth that anyone can be injured by stress. |
| Attitudes of intolerance or even fear of anyone who is different. | Promote an understanding and acceptance of diversity among unit members and their families. Everyone deserves respect. |

## Possible Harm to Career

Organizational stigma is the one that is most tangible and most based on fact—the real harm that can occur to a military career or to future employability because of having been diagnosed and treated for a mental health problem. Applications for security clearances and licensure in a number of fields—from aviation to health care—still include questions asking whether the individual has ever been treated for a mental illness. In most fields, admitting to a mental health history does not immediately disqualify an applicant, but it does trigger a requirement for additional documentation and possibly a current psychiatric evaluation to determine fitness and suitability. Service members whose military and future civilian careers depend on a security clearance or licensure may be highly averse to admitting to anyone that they are experiencing significant stress injury symptoms for fear they will lose important credentials.

For other duties in the Department of Defense that do not require a special clearance or license, written regulations and directives do not specifically state that a mental health diagnosis or treatment should alone determine the employment fitness or suitability of a Service member. The disqualifying factors are based on defects in required capabilities, judgment, reliability, or stability, regardless of how they arise. Physical standards for retention in all Services are broadly defined with few specific disqualifying conditions, so that commanders retain maximum authority to determine the fitness and deployability of Service members based on the capabilities and performance of each individual and not labels they have been given.

The Assistant Secretary of Defense for Health Affairs published a policy memorandum on 07 Nov 2006, *Policy Guidance for Deployment-Limiting Psychiatric Conditions and Medications*, to address questions regarding the deployability to war zones of Service members who had been treated for a mental disorder or who were currently taking a psychiatric medication. This memorandum directed that commanders determine the deployability of Service members on a case-by-case basis after considering all available information. With few exceptions (see chap. 6 for more detail), Service members who are able to perform their assigned duties, are medically stable, and are not a danger to themselves or others should be considered fit and suitable for worldwide deployment regardless of their psychiatric diagnoses.

Real risks to the careers of Marines and Sailors posed by mental health labels must be acknowledged and addressed. Commanders can minimize the impact of this source of mental health stigma by deciding fitness and deployability in every case based solely on proven performance and capabilities, after carefully weighing the risks and benefits of continued service and deployment, rather than on any particular diagnostic label. Commanders can communicate their policies regarding the continued service of Marines or Sailors who have received treatment for a mental health problem. By educating all members of the unit about continued service after mental health treatment, including the very low likelihood of medical or administrative discharge solely because of having sought and accepted help, commanders can defeat the stigma-promoting rumors and distortions that are common among Service members.

## Intolerance for Weakness of Any Kind

The second source of mental health stigma in the military is as ancient as the warrior mindset from which it springs—an admiration for strength in body, mind, and spirit, and a similar intolerance for weakness of any kind. Peer attitudes about strength and weakness are necessary for individuals and units in the military to perform challenging missions under difficult conditions. These same attitudes, however, can cause significant and unintended harm if they prevent individuals from admitting to themselves or others that they are wounded, injured, or ill for fear of appearing weak. The wish to avoid any appearance of weakness can motivate Service members to hide not only their stress symptoms, but also their physical health problems. Marines and Sailors sometimes suffer silently through entire deployments or underway periods with serious, untreated medical problems because they don't want to complain, seem unreliable, or be removed from their units. This unwillingness to accept any sign of weakness in oneself or others may cause health problems that might have been treated easily and quickly in their early stages to become more severe and chronic because they were left untreated. Small problems can become big problems that affect the individual's health and the unit's readiness.

Commanders and other leaders can attack an intolerance of weakness by reminding Marines and Sailors at every opportunity that anyone at any time can be wounded, injured, or become ill, regardless of how well-trained and motivated they are. No one is immune to physical or psychological injury. Though it may hurt one's pride to admit injury to others—especially in a situation from which others walked away unscathed—the greater proof of strength is to have the moral courage to face problems honestly and get the help needed. If Marines or Sailors are reluctant to get help for physical or psychological problems for themselves, they should do it for those who depend on them. Leaders at all levels should also continually monitor their Marines and Sailors for signs of unrecognized or unreported health problems and encourage the buddy system of watching out for each other.

## Belief That Stress Problems Only Happen to the Weak

The common belief that only individuals who are weak in either character or motivation can develop disabling stress symptoms on a battlefield or other extreme operational setting dates back to the early years of World War I. Prior to 1916, military leaders and medical experts around the world believed that combat stress casualties were caused by unseen damage to the brain. During the American Civil War and the beginning of World War I, there was relatively little shame attached to being diagnosed with "nostalgia" or "shell shock" and, given the great intensity of combat in both these wars, many soldiers sought treatment for these problems. Attitudes and beliefs about the nature and causes of combat stress casualties changed abruptly in September 1916 when a group of German psychiatrists in Munich decided by majority vote that shell shock—or *nervenshock* in German—was not caused by literal damage to the brain, but by a pre-existing character weakness known as "hysteria."

This vote was not unanimous because strong scientific evidence existed on both sides of the debate. Those who argued that stress casualties were due to pre-existing personal weakness pointed to the failure of medical science to find any evidence of neurological damage in these patients. They also pointed out that a number of stress casualties were later found to never have been anywhere near an explosive blast at the time their symptoms began and that many stress casualty patients recovered from the physical manifestations of their illnesses, such as paralysis or the loss of vision or hearing, after a course of treatment using only hypnosis or electric shock.

Experts on the other side of the debate argued that soldiers who became stress casualties during combat often had no history of problems coping with stress prior to their military service that would suggest a pre-existing weakness or vulnerability to stress. They also pointed to the growing number of proven brain disorders discovered by medical science that could produce symptoms somewhat similar to those of shell shock or other acute stress injury. These included infections, head injuries, and the effects of ingested substances, such as alcohol. Furthermore, "cures" by hypnosis or the application of electric shock were often only temporary.

Medical science in the early 20th century, like that of today, was incapable of resolving this debate. Under ordinary circumstances, medical professionals would not end a vigorous scientific debate by taking a vote in which the majority view would thereafter be taken to be the "truth" because majority opinions and fact are often not the same. September 1916, however, was not an ordinary time in Germany given the enormous costs to the German Empire of paying soldiers' disability compensation, treating *nervenshock* cases in hospitals, and finding replacements for all the young men evacuated from the front lines as stress casualties.

The historical evidence strongly suggests, according to *Hysterical Men: War, Psychiatry, and the Politics of Trauma in Germany, 1890–1930*, that the vote in Munich in 1916 was taken partly for economic and political reasons, rather than scientific. History also suggests that the label used to describe the pre-existing weakness believed to underlie stress casualties— hysteria—was deliberately chosen to produce shame in the young men given that label. Hysteria literally meant "disturbances of the uterus;" even uneducated young European men in 1916 knew that being compared to a female reproductive organ was feminizing and shameful.

Subsequent to September 1916, militaries on both sides of the war changed their policies about stress casualties. Thereafter, "hysteria" cases were not evacuated from the front lines unless all efforts to restore them to combat duty failed. Those who did not recover were denied further treatment or disability compensation. In the short run, this new policy worked. The greatly increased stigma attached to stress problems made it less likely that soldiers would walk into a battalion aid station requesting help. Those who did reach a medical care center were less likely to be evacuated to the rear, so epidemics of stress casualties quickly abated. In the long run, however, the view that only individuals with pre-existing weakness could become stress casualties failed to solve the combat stress problem and, in some ways, made it worse.

During World War II, massive efforts to screen out those with pre-existing weakness prior to induction failed to reduce the rates of psychiatric casualties in the military services of any nation, in any theater of war. The enhanced burden of stigma associated with mental health problems in the military also erected barriers to psychological treatment that continue today.

Modern military leaders may be reluctant to take steps to reduce the stigma caused by equating stress problems with weakness for fear of reigniting stress epidemics similar to those of the Civil War or World War I. This logic fails to take several crucial factors into account. The military's current problem is not an excessive willingness on the part of Marines and Sailors to come forward requesting help for stress problems. It is, instead, a deep-seated reluctance to admit to having stress or mental health problems of any kind, either during or after deployment.

Medical and psychological sciences have advanced greatly since 1916; current treatments for stress injuries and illnesses tend to be far more effective and successful in most cases if the individual accepts treatment. The current mission of the US military—to fight a long war on multiple fronts with an all volunteer force—demands that military personnel resources be tightly conserved. Hence, identifying and treating all health problems early so full functional capacity can be restored as quickly as possible is an important means toward that end. The core values of the Navy and Marine Corps require that their commitment to the welfare of Sailors, Marines, and their family members not falter because they have been damaged by the stress of military service. Education and awareness is the best way to fight the stigma arising from the misconception that stress and mental health problems arise only in those with pre-existing weakness.

## Intolerance or Fear of Those Different From Oneself

People are naturally most comfortable being in the company of others who are similar to them in appearance, attitudes, and behavior. Likewise, many are most uncomfortable, ill at ease, or fearful of others who differ from them in important ways. This aspect of human nature, while not negative, has resulted in many negative and destructive attitudes and behaviors over the course of human history. Frequent targets of intolerance, based on appearing different, have been individuals with noticeable disabilities, such as those who are missing limbs, paralyzed, or unable to speak or to hear normally. The number of derogatory words in our language that refer to such individuals, including the common and generic term "cripple," is testimony to the stigma to which they have been subjected.

Our society has successfully fought such stigma through legislation, education, and other means. For example, at the time that President Franklin Delano Roosevelt became paralyzed by polio, in the early 1920s, it was still very common for paralytics to be openly jeered and ridiculed in public settings—and not only by children. Through Roosevelt's leadership and advocacy for those afflicted with polio, it soon became unthinkable to laugh at a person's disability.

Individuals who have been injured by stress or who suffer from stress illnesses, such as PTSD, are not crippled, but the discomfort certain individuals feel when in the presence of someone with a stress injury or PTSD can be very similar to that associated with any other condition that makes someone different. Those who have never been damaged by stress often cannot imagine how or why those with stress injuries behave the way they do. No amount of description can bridge that gap in understanding, as, in the same way, someone who has never had polio cannot understand the plight of President Roosevelt and the millions of others afflicted with that disease. Leaders attack intolerance most effectively by setting an example of tolerance and respect for diversity, even when it is hard to understand, and through education and setting and enforcing standards of mutual respect and tolerance. There is no reason why the stigma associated with stress and mental health problems should not be replaced with the same degree of compassion and empathy with which most physical injuries and illnesses are now treated.

# Combat and Operational Stress First Aid

First aid is a set of procedures for the initial premedical care of injuries and illnesses. The first time in history procedures for the initial care of physical injuries and illnesses were practiced in a systematic way was during the 11th century, as a method for military personnel to care for their own combat casualties in the field. The earliest practitioners of combat first aid were warriors of the Order of St. John, Knights of Malta, established in 1080 AD.

First aid principles and practices saw a decline during the Dark Ages; however, in the mid-20<sup>th</sup> century, the first International Geneva Convention established the International Red Cross Society specifically to promote humane and timely care of sick and injured soldiers in the field. More recently, these same principles of physical first aid, developed over the centuries, have also been applied to the premedical care of injuries and illnesses in civilians.

The paragraphs that follow describe the core actions of COS first aid, hereafter called "stress first aid." Stress first aid was developed by the Marine Corps, Navy, and the National Center for PTSD, building on earlier psychological first aid (PFA) tools created for first responders to civilian accidents and disasters. Stress first aid differs from PFA in that it is specifically intended for use in units and families of the Navy and Marine Corps, in military settings from the training field to the battlefield, and from home to the office. It is an ongoing process rather than a one-shot intervention and follows the stress continuum model.

Just like first aid for physical injuries and illnesses, stress first aid is a set of tools with three aims—to preserve life, prevent further harm, and promote recovery. The types of life-threat and harm that stress first aid address are very different from those targeted by physical first aid as are the methods employed, but the intended outcomes are the same.

Neither physical first aid nor stress first aid is intended to take the place of prevention efforts or medical or surgical care when that is needed. In actuality, they serve as temporary measures in preparation for more definitive treatment when it is indicated and to increase the probability of the success of such treatment when it becomes available. In many cases of more mild injury or illness, first aid or stress first aid may be all that is required to preserve life, prevent further damage, and promote recovery.

In the case of physical injuries and illnesses, prevention efforts can take the form of health promotion procedures, personal protective equipment, or physical readiness standards. In the case of stress injuries and illnesses, prevention takes many forms, including those aimed at strengthening and mitigating stress.

Stress first aid requires a set of skills designed to address a certain type of problem in a certain situation—the ability to perform a quick and accurate assessment, to find the best way to meet the specific needs indentified, and to identify when more than first aid

---

**Goals of Stress First Aid**

Preserve life.

Prevent further harm.

Promote recovery.

---

**Skills Needed for Stress First Aid**

Access quickly.

Match response to need.

Ensure further treatment.

---

is needed to ensure that such further treatment is received quickly. These skills require familiarity with the many signs and symptoms of injury and the uses and limitations of resources available. Flexibility is the key, since each situation is unique. Stress first aid consists of seven actions and is organized on three levels—

- Continuous Aid.
  - Check.
  - Coordinate.
- Primary Aid.
  - Cover.
  - Calm.
- Secondary Aid.
  - Connect.
  - Competence.
  - Confidence.

Each of these seven actions—the seven Cs of stress first aid (see fig. 5-1 on page 5-12 and table 5-2 on page 5-13)—is described in the following sections, along with examples of specific situations in which each particular action might best be used. As an initial orientation, it is helpful to understand the three levels of stress first aid—continuous, primary, and secondary—and how they differ.

Continuous aid includes the two stress first aid actions, check and coordinate, to be considered by leaders of Marines and Sailors all the time. Navy and Marine Corps leaders must continuously assess and reassess the stress zones of unit and family members in order to know who is at risk and who is in need of treatment or other care. Leaders must also continuously make judgments about what additional resources or referrals may be needed by their Sailors or Marines in order to master the challenges they face and recover from stress reactions, injuries, or illnesses.

Primary aid includes the two stress first aid actions of cover and calm. These two actions can be taken by anyone in almost any situation. Everyone in the military, including family members, should be familiar with them. Cover and calm should also be considered first when responding to a stress injury in another person or in oneself and are typically only used briefly in situations of intense distress or losses of function.

Secondary aid includes the last three stress first aid actions of connect, competence, and confidence. These secondary aid actions should be considered once it is clear that either the primary aid actions of cover and calm are no longer needed or they were never needed at all. The secondary aid actions tend to be more the responsibility of military leaders and their religious ministry and medical support personnel than the two primary aid actions. Furthermore, secondary aid actions tend to be needed over a longer period of time during the process of recovering from a stress injury or illness.

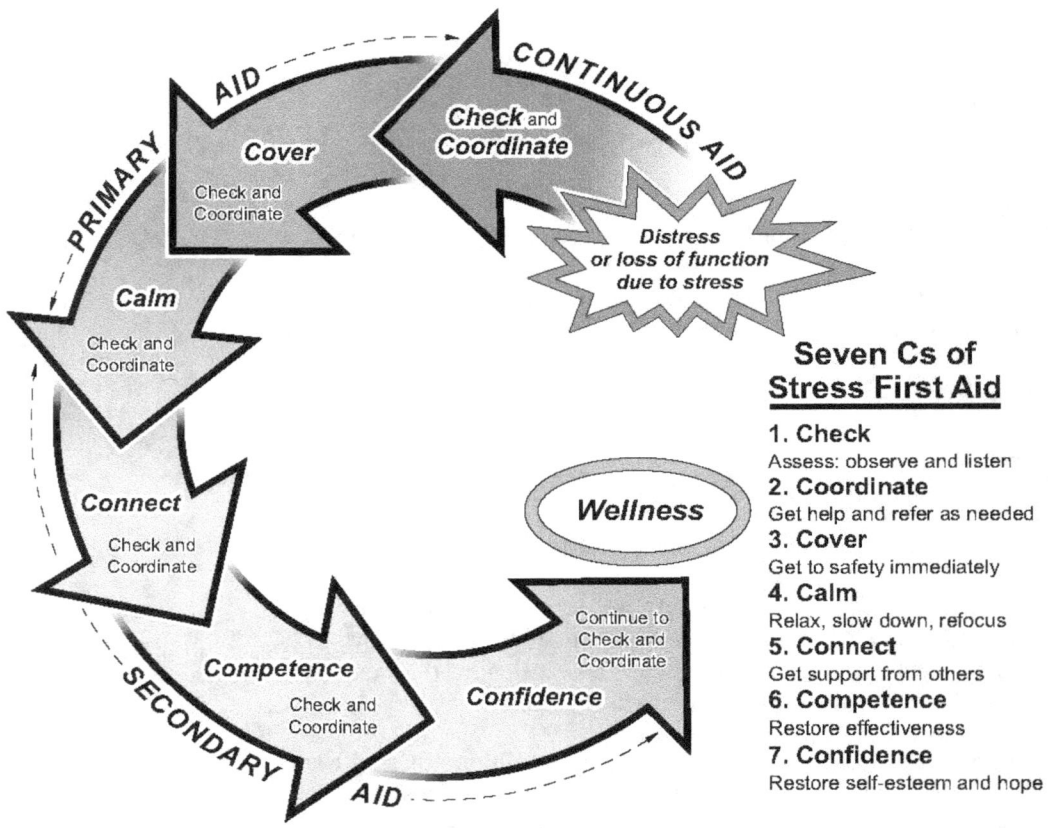

**Figure 5-1.** Stress First Aid.

Table 5-2. Overview of Stress First Aid.

| | Goals | When It Is Used | How You Do It |
|---|---|---|---|
| **Check** | Identify stress zone and need for stress first aid. Assess effectiveness of stress first aid actions. Monitor recovery. | After every significant stressor. After applying stress first aid. After every deployment. Whenever needed, repeatedly and often. | Watch and listen for: Unusual stressors. Severe distress. Changes in normal functioning or behavior. |
| **Coordinate** | Inform others who need to know. Refer for additional help. Make sure help is received. | Every time significant stress problems are identified. Whenever needed, repeatedly and often. | Inform chain of command (one level up). Refer to care provider, if indicated. Follow through. |
| **Cover** | Get individual to safety as soon as possible. Prevent others from being harmed. | Briefly, when stressed persons are at risk or place others at risk until mental focus and self-control return. | Recognize danger posed by or to a stressed person. Neutralize the danger. Keep person safe until he recovers. |
| **Calm** | Reduce heart rate. Reduce emotional intensity. Regain mental focus. | When a person's level of physical activation or emotions are too intense for a situation. | Stop activity and relax. Slow, deep breathing. Refocus thinking. Use "grounding" techniques. |
| **Connect** | Promote peer support. Prevent stressed individuals from isolating themselves. | When stressful events cause loss of trust, respect, and communication in unit or family. | Spend time with stressed persons. Ask how they are doing. Encourage peer support. |
| **Competence** | Restore mental and physical capabilities. Restore role functioning. | Stress injury or illness causes loss or change in normal functioning and abilities. | Encourage and mentor back to full function, step by step. Retrain, if necessary. |
| **Confidence** | Restore self-confidence. Restore self-esteem. Restore hope. | Any time an individual loses confidence in self, peers, leaders, or equipment. | Provide experiences of mastery. Positive reinforcement. Increasing responsibility. |

## Continuous Aid
## Actions of Stress First Aid

The two continuous aid actions—check and coordinate—are so integral to the ongoing health and well-being of Service members that the other five Cs won't work without them. They are the backbone that supports the rest of the skeleton.

### Check

The check action of stress first aid includes continuous reassessment of the effects and outcomes of other actions taken, such as is included in the familiar plan-do-check-act cycle.

*What is it?* At its most basic level, the check action of stress first aid is the process of assessing a Marine, Sailor, or family member for his current stress zone, as described in chapter 4. Identifying stress zones may be only the first of many steps of assessment in stress first aid. In cases in which an Orange Zone stress injury or Red Zone stress illness are deemed present, further assessment must be carried out by leaders or caregivers to determine what next actions must be taken to preserve life, prevent further harm, and promote recovery. Similar to the assessment and application of physical first aid, it is not enough to know merely that an individual has been injured. To really be helpful, one must assess the nature and severity of the injury and what specific threats to life and safety must also be addressed.

*Who does it?* The check action is the responsibility of everyone in the military. The hierarchy of shared responsibility in the Navy commonly summarized in the sequence, "ship, shipmates, self" can be applied to the check action of stress first aid. All individuals have a responsibility to continuously check shipmates, family members, friends, and themselves for signs that other actions may be needed.

*In which situations might it be used?* There are no limitations to the situations in which the check action is both appropriate and necessary.

*How is it done?* The check action in stress first aid is performed in much the same way as stress zones are identified, by watching and listening for key indicators of distress or alterations in normal functioning. All available information must be considered.

The goals of the check action of stress first aid are—

- Identify stress zone.
- Recognize need for stress first aid.
- Decide which specific actions are needed.
- Evaluate outcome of actions taken.

## Coordinate

The coordinate action is always more than merely a hand off to someone else; it is good leadership.

*What is it?* The coordinate component of stress first aid includes many different actions a military leader might take on behalf of a Marine or Sailor recovering from a stress injury or illness. The common feature of all coordinate functions is that they make other people aware of the problems at hand or bring other resources to bear on them. Any others who might be made aware of or resources that might be recruited to help address a stress problem depend on the level of the leader and the nature of the problem. In the case of a petty officer or junior NCO using stress first aid to help a unit member, one form of coordination might be informing other members of the chain of command about the acute stress problems that have become apparent. In this case, a petty officer or NCO should ask the question, "Who else needs to know?" To determine what other resources might be obtained to help a Service member or family member recover from a stress injury or illness, the pertinent question to ask is, "Who else can help?" The answer to that question could include chaplains, medical specialists, mental health counselors, and representatives of any of dozens of available personnel and wellness services. Coordination requires ongoing follow-up to ensure that the right people continue to be aware and involved and that needed services are being received.

*Who does it?* Like the check action, coordination is the responsibility of everyone in the military; however, small unit leaders at the petty officer and NCO level bear the greatest responsibility for the coordinate action. Family members and individual Service members may also perform needed coordinate actions.

*In which situations might it be used?* There are no limitations to the situations in which the coordinate action is both appropriate and necessary.

*How is it done?* The coordinate action requires all the skills of a small unit leader, "at the deck plates" and "boots on the ground." Communication and perseverance are keys to success.

The goals of the coordinate action of stress first aid are—

- Inform others of a unit member's stress problem.
- Bring in additional help.
- Make sure needed help is obtained.

## Primary Aid Actions of Stress First Aid

The two primary aid actions, cover and calm, are grouped together because they have two features in common—they are both tools designed to be used only briefly, at moments of the greatest distress, or when functioning is altered because of stress. They are both simple enough to be performed by one person taking care of his own stress symptoms or by any one person rendering stress first aid to another. These two actions comprise self-aid and buddy aid for stress. Cover and calm are primary aid actions because they should always be considered first before moving on to anything else. Cover and calm can be lifesaving, prevent further harm, and promote recovery.

### Cover

Cover is short for "get to cover" or "take cover," which means to get to safety.

*What is it?* The cover action applies only to situations in which individuals may be in danger and their ability to effectively perceive and manage that danger is compromised because of a stress reaction, injury, or illness. Being in a dangerous situation does not warrant a stress first aid action, such as cover. Rather, the need for the cover action of stress first aid as a potentially life-saving intervention is defined by the relative inability of a particular individual at a particular moment in time to fully appreciate the danger he faces or to respond appropriately to it because of stress. Dangerous situations that might require the cover action of stress first aid include the full range of military operations, from taking incoming fire on a battlefield to operating dangerous equipment, such as the catapult on the deck of an aircraft carrier. They also include situations in which the immediate threat is nonmilitary, such as driving or walking in traffic or handling cutlery in a galley. The key indicator of need for the cover action of stress first aid is that an individual is unable to as accurately perceive and effectively respond to threats to his own or others' safety as he would normally, specifically because of the distress or changes in functioning that accompany a stress reaction, injury, or illness.

*Who does it?* Anyone in the military or in military families may be called upon to perform the cover action of stress first aid. Situations in which it may be necessary tend to develop very quickly, often with little time to get help from anyone else. Cover actions must be performed by the closest person, often a buddy, shipmate, or family member. Cover actions tend to be much more effective if they are performed by persons who are known and trusted by the individual experiencing severe stress. A stress-induced loss of ability to fully comprehend an imminent life-threat may make it difficult for an individual to appreciate that a person is helping them. The cover action of stress first aid may also be performed by stress-injured individuals for their own benefit as a first step in stress self-aid. Cover is the most basic form of stress self-aid or buddy aid.

*In which situation might it be used?* There are three types of situations in which cover might be needed and used—when a person jeopardizes his own safety because he is unable to appropriately think and react to external threats; when a stress-injured person places others in added jeopardy because of his mental state; and when a stress-injured or ill person is in danger not because of external threats but because of internal reasons, such as thoughts of suicide. In all such dangerous situations, the most appropriate cover action is usually the one that neutralizes the threat least intrusively. Possible cover actions include both verbal and nonverbal interventions, ranging from a simple verbal warning to physically taking control of the other person. Appendix F is a list of a few of the ways in which a stress injury may affect an individual's behavior and ability to manage current threats. Table 5-3 lists examples of dangerous situations in which a cover action might be required, along with possible cover actions appropriate to each situation.

*How is it done?* Specific leader actions that fall under the heading of cover vary greatly from situation to situation, depending on the nature of the immediate threat and the degree to which an individual is unable to manage that threat. As in any other intervention that potentially limits another person's independent decisionmaking and freedom, the least restrictive measure is usually the best, as long as safety is ensured. At one end of the

**Table 5-3.** Examples of Siutations in Which Cover Actions Might be Required.

| Situation | Possible Cover Actions |
|---|---|
| A ground combat Marine suddenly goes blank and becomes unresponsive during a firefight. | If necessary, a nearby person physically pulls Marine to a safe position and holds him there. |
| | If Marine can respond to voice commands, nearby person gives Marine simple directions regarding what to do next. |
| | Nearby person ensures Marine's weapon is being used safely. |
| A Sailor working on antennas in the superstructure of a ship suddenly becomes immobile and begins to shake and cling to whatever is nearby. | Nearby shipmate or supervisor uses verbal encouragement to help Sailor stay calm and to decide what to do. |
| | If Sailor responds to voice commands, give him simple directions regarding how to get to a safe position. |
| | If necessary, shipmate or supervisor physically assists Sailor down from superstructure. |
| A deployed Marine, who had recently been acting strange and withdrawn from others, inappropriately sets his weapon to Condition 1 and walks out of a berthing area at night without saying a word. | Nearby unit members accompany Marine to determine his intentions. |
| | They encourage Marine to return his weapon to the appropriate condition. |
| | If necessary, they take physical control of the Marine and his weapon. |
| An intoxicated military spouse begins waving a kitchen knife while engaged in an angry dispute with her husband at home. | Husband or friends calmly but persistently urge military spouse to put the knife down. |
| | If necessary, police are called to further ensure safety. |
| The driver of a vehicle in a war zone at night reacts to the nearby detonation of an IED by accelerating to an unnecessary and unsafe speed after turning off the vehicle's headlights. | Vehicle commander uses simple voice commands to urge driver to reduce speed and take other action as required. |
| | If necessary, vehicle commander stops vehicle. |
| After witnessing the death of a close friend during a firefight, a Marine blindly charges an enemy position while screaming. | If time permits, others nearby give Marine verbal commands to stop. |
| | If necessary, others nearby tackle Marine and physically pull him back to a safe position. |
| A Navy SEAL has a vivid recollection onf a recent combat action triggered by smells in a restaurant while on liberty with his family and he announces his intent to retrieve the loaded pistol he keeps in his car. | Spouse or friends in attendance verbally discourage Navy SEAL from retrieving his weapon. |
| | If necessary, others accompany SEAL to ensure his safety while urging him not to retrieve weapon. |
| | If necessary, police are called to further ensure safety. |
| Legend SEAL—sea-air-land team | |

spectrum, the cover action of stress first aid is nothing less than physically taking control of another person to prevent him from harming himself or someone else or to get him out of harm's way. At the other end of the spectrum, cover might be nothing more than a suggestion or nudge to help a stressed individual effectively evaluate and manage a dangerous situation.

## Calm

The calm action of stress first aid is the natural partner to the cover action. Situations that require a cover action will almost always also require a calm action, either simultaneously or immediately afterward.

*What is it?* Calming is the process by which individuals experiencing intense distress or alterations in functioning because of stress reactions, injuries, or illnesses are helped to reduce the intensity of their physical and emotional responses to perceived dangerous situations and to regain mental focus and control. The importance to both health and safety of promptly reducing excessive levels of physical and emotional activation in high stress situations cannot be overstated. Calming is crucial because the brain's ability to function is optimal only in a relatively narrow range of levels of physical activation. At levels above or below that optimal range, the ability of the brain to process information and the mind's ability to think clearly, make rational decisions, and control impulses, falls off sharply. For example, a person whose level of physical activation is very low because he just woke up or is very tired and sleepy is not capable of thinking as quickly and sharply as someone who is fully alert and mobilized. So, too, a person whose level of physical and emotional activation is too high because he has just been injured by a life-threat stressor, for example, is also not as capable of thinking, deciding, and acting as the person whose level of activation is in the optimal range. Although each individual is unique, heart rate is a good indicator of a person's level of physical activation. For example, if an individual operates best with a heart rate of 130 times per minute, that person almost certainly will not be able to think and act as well with a heart rate of 180 beats per minute. Therefore, if someone's mental processes have been degraded because of excessive physical activation, then slowing down the heart rate and other indicators of activation will always improve mental performance. Calming is also crucial to health and safety because the risk for biological damage or even the death of nerve cells in the brain is directly proportional to the level of physical activation. The higher the heart rate, the greater the risk that a given stressor situation will inflict an injury to important control

> Quickly reducing the level of physical activation, such as by slowing heart rate, and calming emotional intensity can save the mind and brain from further damage from stress.

circuits in the brain. The lower the heart rate, the lower the risk, so reducing the level of physical activation when it is excessive for a given situation is like putting out a fire before it can do any more damage. The calm action of stress first aid targets not only heart rate, but also intense emotions, such as excessive fear or anger, that can interfere with rational decisionmaking and self-control.

*Who does it?* Like the cover action of stress first aid, the calm action is often required in situations that develop rapidly and resolve almost as rapidly. Just as with the cover action, anyone can be called upon to perform the calm action of stress first aid, either for himself or for someone else. Everyone in the military should be skilled in the use of the calming techniques described in appendix J, *Calming and Focusing Techniques.*

*In which situation might it be used?* The calm action is appropriate in any situation in which an individual's level of physical or emotional activation is excessive for that situation. Military leaders do not need to keep track of their unit members' heart rates in order to recognize situations requiring calming actions; instead, they can observe the distress and loss of normal physical and mental function that accompany the excessive activation levels resulting from Orange Zone stress injuries or Red Zone stress illnesses, such as PTSD. In those situations in which an immediate threat to safety is present, the calm action will be appropriate either with or immediately after the cover action. In situations that do not include an immediate threat, the calm action is performed without delay.

*How is it done?* The calm action can be performed through a number of techniques, ranging in complexity from simple physical presence, such as remaining silently near an individual experiencing severe stress, to the practicing of a set of specific procedures designed to reduce heart rate or promote the return of mental focus and control. Anything that works is worth doing. A common feature of all effective calming actions is that they require the person doing the calming to also be calm. Among medical treatment personnel, this principle is sometimes stated as, "First, take your own pulse." The point is to remain calm while trying to aid others. Screaming at someone who is on the verge of losing control because of stress does not help.

The goals of the calm action of stress first aid are—

- Reduce the level of physical activation, such as heart rate.
- Reduce intensity of negative emotions, such as fear or anger.
- Regain mental focus and control.

## Secondary Aid
## Actions of Stress First Aid

The three secondary aid actions—connect, competence, and confidence—are grouped together because they have several features in common. First, these actions are not typically taken during the earliest stages of response to an Orange Zone stress injury. Rather, they are employed after the initial threats to safety have passed and the stress-injured individual has become more like his usual self. Second, these three secondary aid actions are much more the responsibility of leaders and caregivers than are the two primary aid actions and are not self-aid or buddy aid. Finally, these three actions tend to be employed over a longer period of time than the two primary aid actions, since the need for them does not disappear as soon as the initial stress injury symptoms abate.

### Connect

The connect action of stress first aid can be thought of as intentionally using unit cohesion for the benefit of stress-injured Marines or Sailors in the unit. The connect action can also be thought of as repairing unit cohesion, since cohesion is almost always damaged in a unit that experiences significant life-threat, loss, or inner-conflict stress.

*What is it?* The connect action of stress first aid can be described most simply as ensuring peer support for those recovering from Orange Zone stress injuries or Red Zone stress illnesses. No specific form of social support is required. For example, the stress-injured person does not need to recount the vivid details of his experiences of life-threat or loss as is required of psychological debriefing procedures. Rather, the connect action is merely the absence of social isolation, since social alienation obstructs healing from stress injuries and makes symptoms worse over time instead of better. Social support is as important to the healing of a stress wound as a bandage or splint is to the healing of a wound to the muscle and bone of a limb. The connect action of stress first aid is closely related to unit cohesion, an important component of the strengthen COSC and OSC leadership function. Both unit cohesion and the social support needed to promote healing from a stress injury require attitudes of mutual trust, respect, and communication within the unit. Stress-injured Marines and Sailors almost always withdraw from those around them and lose some of the trust and camaraderie they had previously enjoyed. The connect action of stress first aid must address and repair such losses of unit cohesion. An important tool for all military leaders in performing the connect action of stress first aid is the unit AAR, as described in appendix E. An AAR can be a vehicle for a unit leader to actively promote and repair both horizontal and vertical communication in a unit of any size. It can also help discover and remove obstacles to mutual trust and respect arising from Orange Zone stress.

*Who does it?* Every member of a unit can contribute both to unit cohesion and to the social support needed to recover from a stress injury. Every family member contributes to these same functions in families. Though unit religious ministry and medical support personnel can be particularly helpful in developing and maintaining connectedness in a unit affected by severe stress, the ultimate responsibility for the connect action always resides with the commander.

*In which situation might it be used?* Table 5-4 provides examples of situations in which the connect action of stress first aid might be important.

*How is it done?* The simplest and most direct method of connecting with a Marine or Sailor who has just experienced an intense stressor, such as a life-threat or loss, is to approach him in a nonthreatening, casual manner and strike up a conversation. Even if no words are spoken about the recent stressful experience, the Marine or Sailor will get the message that they are valued. During the course of that conversation, the simple words, "How are you doing?" or "Are you OK?" can also be reassuring, even if the Marine or Sailor does not feel able to talk about it. If a stress-injured person wishes to talk about his experiences, then listening without passing judgment will almost certainly help. The person should not be forced to talk about the incident or even asked to describe the details unless interested in doing so.

The goals of the connect action of stress first aid are—

- Don't allow stress-injured individuals to withdraw from others.
- Promote positive peer support.
- Restore mutual trust and respect.

**Table 5-4.** Examples of Situations in Which Connect Actions Might be Required.

| Situation | Possible Connect Actions |
|---|---|
| A squadron aircraft crashes, killing all aboard. Rumors suggest that poor maintenance was at fault. Squadron aircrew personnel avoid speaking or interacting with maintenance personnel. Squadron cohesion falls. | Conduct AARs in small units, such as work centers, both to learn what happened and to increase communication. Attack rumors with fact. Share the blame. Encourage trust and respect. |
| Young ground combat Marine freezes during his first firefight in Afghanistan. Although only disabled for a few seconds, he feels ashamed and withdraws from all contact with other unit members. | AARs at squad or fire team level are not to put the young Marine on the spot but to put into perspective what happened—what harm, if any, did the young Marine's freezing do? One-on-one mentorship of the young Marine by more senior Marines willing to admit to their own stress in the past. |
| A Navy SEABEE unit is extended in Iraq beyond the 12 months originally scheduled for its deployment. Some unit members believe their commanding officer unnecessarily volunteered them to extend their deployment. Communication up and down the chain of command slows and trust in leadership diminishes. | Unit commander may communicate to unit members the reasons for the deployment extension and what purpose will be served by the unit during the remainder of their deployment. AARs in small units to reinforce peer support. |
| A Marine driver of a HMMWV in a combat zone accidentally hits and kills another Marine while operating his vehicle in the dark with all running lights turned off, as directed by the vehicle commander. The driver of the vehicle blames himself completely for the accidental death. He withdraws from social interaction with others in his unit. | Small unit leaders and trusted peers do not let HMMWV driver isolate himself. AARs to discuss the accident at the small unit level, including ways to prevent a recurrence. More senior Marines mentor young driver to forgive himself. Blame is shared by all who contributed, so the accident is no one person's fault |
| Legend:<br>HMMWV–high mobility multipurpose wheeled vehicle<br>SEABEE–Navy construction engineer | |

# Competence

Competence is really short for "help restore previous capabilities" or "cultivate personal competence."

*What is it?* The need for this action of stress first aid is signaled by the loss of previous mental, emotional, or physical capabilities directly because of an Orange Zone stress injury or Red Zone stress illness. Which capabilities may be lost and to what extent will depend greatly on the situation and the individual involved. For certain individuals at certain times, Orange Zone stress may cause no discernible loss of mental or physical abilities. On the other hand, a severe life-threat or loss injury may cause a brief period of significant mental confusion followed by a longer period of slightly decreased ability to think clearly and sharply or to control intense emotions. Such mild changes in capabilities are almost always accompanied by somewhat larger losses in self-confidence and trust in one's own abilities. The competence action of stress first aid aims to restore the confidence in previous mental and physical capabilities through practicing them and demonstrating effectiveness. The critical role that leaders play in this process is to encourage and mentor the re-establishment of important mental and physical capabilities.

*Who does it?* The competence action of stress first aid is largely the responsibility of small unit leaders at the level of petty officer or NCO, although peers and family members also participate in this action.

*In which situations might it be used?* Table 5-5 lists examples of situations in which the competence action may be appropriate.

*How is it done?* The competence action of stress first aid, as a means to promote recovery from a stress injury, is analogous to physical therapy to promote recovery from a limb injury, such as a severe sprain or fracture. As the underlying injury heals, full function will not return unless the injured part is required to perform the function for which it was designed, sometimes with gradually increasing intensity over a period of time. The competence action of stress first aid is similar, except that the injured part is not an arm or leg, but the mind and breain. Mentorship and leadership are crucial to the process of recovering lost functions, just as a good physical therapist is crucial to recovering lost limb function after a sprain or fracture. Other crucial components of the competence action, as described in table 5-5, are a continual reassessment of capabilities in collaboration with medical and mental health professionals as the Service member returns to work and regular feedback on progress is made.

The goals of the competence action of stress first aid are—

- Restore mental capabilities.
- Restore physical capabilities.
- Restore trust in those capabilities.

Table 5-5. Examples of Situations in Which Competence Actions Might be Required.

| Situation | Possible Competence Actions |
|---|---|
| Marine or Sailor with a significant life-threat stress injury briefly experiences persistent mental confusion and slowed, unclear thinking. | Require the Marine or Sailor to gradually resume responsibility for doing work that requires clear thinking, planning, and decisionmaking.<br><br>Continually reassess mental capacity and give the Marine or Sailor regular feedback on progress. |
| Petty officer or NCO who developed a wear-and-tear stress injury over long and repeated deployments loses the ability to stay emotionally calm when dealing with subordinates. | As the petty officer or NCO heals from the wear-and-tear stress injury, gradually increase the responsibility he has for subordinates.<br><br>Continually reassess ability to remain emotionally calm under stress and give regular feedback. |
| Small unit leader who loses a member of the unit becomes unable to send subordinates into hazardous situations without worrying excessively about their safety. | As the small unit leader heals from the loss stress injury, gradually increase his responsibility for subordinates being exposed to dangers. Continually reassess ability to refrain from worrying and give regular feedback. |
| Marine or Sailor with severe life-threat stress injury is uncharacteristically unable to maintain own hygiene and cleanliness without supervision. | Gradually increase individual's responsibility for his own hygiene and cleanliness. Reassess and give regular feedback. |

## Confidence

Confidence is retored through the painstaking process of realistically challenging an individual's capacities as he heals from a sterss injury and demonstrating to him his own capabilities.

*What it is?* The confidence action of stress first aid also refers to restoring self-confidence, self-esteem, and hope, since one of the consequences of a severe stress injury or illness can be a loss of hope for one's future. Confidence is the capstone of the process of recovering from a stress injury. Individuals who recover from a stress injury sometimes can regain all previous mental and physical capacities and acquire new ones. The acquisition of new capabilities during the process of recovering from a stress injury is sometimes called "posttraumatic growth."

*Who does it?* Leaders who are role models for Marines and Sailors and whose opinions are highly valued are in powerful positions to restore confidence. Spouses and other significant family members are also crucial for promoting the restoration of confidence. In the end, though, the most important people in the confidence action are the individuals recovering from a stress injury or illness. The investments they make in their own health and well-being are the ones that pay the greatest dividends.

*In which situations might it be used?* There are few limitations to the number and variety of situations in which confidence action of stress first aid may be useful. Restoration of confidence is most crucial after an Orange Zone stress injury or Red Zone stress illness has caused an individual to lose self-confidence.

*How is it done?* Realistic self-confidence and self-esteem are earned through mastering challenges and achieving goals despite hardships and obstacles. The role that leaders play in this process is to help stress-injured Sailors and Marines to set realistic goals, and then to achieve them despite the frustrations they are certain to encounter.

The goals of the confidence action of stress first aid are—

* Restore self-confidence.
* Restore self-esteem.
* Restore hope.

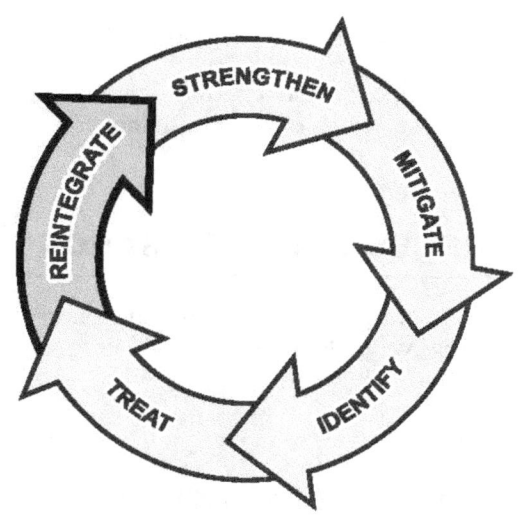

# REINTEGRATE: FIFTH CORE FUNCTION FOR LEADERS

Sailors and Marines are valuable assets and each one possesses a broad base of knowledge, skills, and values learned from their families, schools, and churches prior to entry into military service. Every Service member also possesses unique military-specific capabilities acquired through training and operational experience while in uniform. Every Marine and Sailor is an investment that must be conserved and protected as much as possible. Recruiting and training replacements in the junior ranks is time consuming and expensive, but replacing NCOs and officers of more senior ranks is nearly impossible.

The fifth and final core COSC and OSC function for leaders, reintegrate, focuses directly on the imperative to retain and fully use Sailors and Marines who have been injured by stress and either have recovered or are in the process of recovering. Reintegration includes four key processes for leaders—

- Evaluating and forming judgments about psychological fitness and suitability for duty, including worldwide deployment.
- Assigning Service members who are recovering from stress injuries or illnesses to duties that make the best use of their capabilities.

- Changing whatever attitudes in members of military units that might get in the way of accepting these individuals back in the unit.
- Easing the transition to veteran and civilian status of those Marines and Sailors whose recovery is insufficient to permit return to full duty.

# Addressing the Goals and Challenges of Reintegration

The primary goal of reintegration is to prevent the Navy and Marine Corps from losing valuable personnel. Other goals of reintegration are to—

- Ensure psychological readiness.
- Prevent unnecessary loss of personnel.
- Restore a sense of honor to the psychologically wounded.
- Reduce the stigma associated with treatment.

Reintegration is also part of what the Services consider a sacred duty not to abandon those who have sacrificed a portion of their health and well-being for others; however, it may be one of the most challenging COSC and OSC functions for military leaders because it requires the reconciliation of competing priorities. On one side of the reintegration challenge is the need leaders have to trust that every unit member will perform effectively during every future challenge and perform their assigned roles without limitations. Leaders want all members of their units to be "full up rounds," ready to perform as expected at every moment. If personnel issues were of no concern—if recruits and seasoned veterans were both in limitless supply and the impact on mental health stigma of personnel policies could be ignored—one way to ensure maximum psychological readiness would be to quickly separate from active duty everyone that showed signs of significant distress or loss of normal functioning due to stress. Similarly, maximum physical readiness might best be promoted by immediately separating every Service member who had been physically wounded or injured in any way during an operational deployment. But what would be the consequences of such an extreme policy? What imperatives lie on the other side of the reintegration challenge?

One certain consequence of indiscriminately removing from active duty every Service member identified as having experienced an Orange Zone stress injury or Red Zone stress illness would be the loss of many Sailors and Marines who were still highly capable of serving in the military and contributing to their units' missions either because their original injuries were not too severe or because they had healed sufficiently to return to mission readiness. The same negative outcome would surely follow a policy of indiscriminately discharging every Service member who had been diagnosed and treated for one particular type of physical injury, such as a leg fracture. If each Marine or Sailor who sustained a leg fracture while on active duty was automatically awarded a medical discharge as physically unfit for duty, regardless of how fully the member had recovered or was capable of performing his duties, then many highly fit and fully capable members would be unnecessarily lost from military service forever.

Another very serious negative consequence of such a policy would be an even greater reluctance on the part on Marines and Sailors to acknowledge such stress injuries and to seek help for them. If everyone who sought care for a stress injury were automatically separated from the Service, the only Marines and Sailors who would come forward asking for help would be those who were looking for a way out of the Service or those whose impairment or distress had become so profound they could no longer hide it. Higher barriers to seeking and accepting care would delay treatment for those who need it, probably resulting in greater rates of negative stress-related outcomes, such as divorce, domestic violence, misconduct, substance abuse, suicide, and homicide.

The Navy and Marine Corps can neither afford to in-discriminately separate every Marine and Sailor who suffers a stress injury or illness nor to keep every wounded Service member, regardless of how severe their injuries and disability. The challenge of reintegration for leaders is to find the best balance between the equally unacceptable policies of retaining every Service member who has experienced a stress injury or illness regardless of ongoing functional impairment and risk and indiscriminately discharging every stress-injured Service member regardless of ability to continue to serve. In every case, what should matter is not the type of injury an individual has sustained, but how fully he has recovered and how well he can perform required duties. Every case requires the weighing of specific capabilities against specific limitations.

In the battle against mental health stigma (see fig. 6-1), it is not enough to merely retain individuals on active duty and in an operational unit who prove themselves capable of doing their jobs after recovering from a stress injury or illness. To fully reintegrate such Service members, their leaders and peers must communicate a consistent attitude of respect and trust. They must be given a fair opportunity to fully restore their sense of honor by proving their competence and reclaiming their self-confidence. Given the sometimes insidious nature of negative attitudes about stress injuries held by some Service members, creating an environment in which those recovering from stress can regain the respect and trust of their peers and leaders can be another great challenge for military leaders.

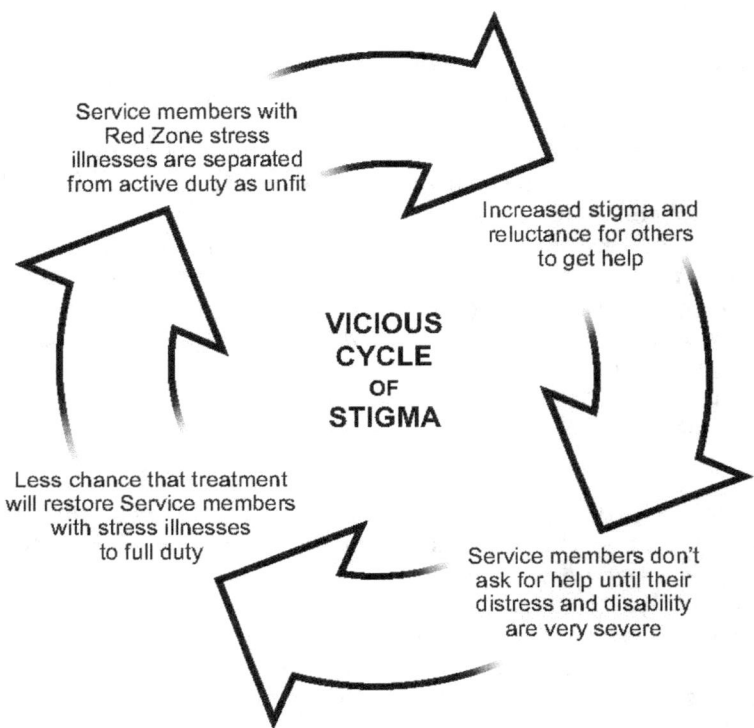

**Figure 6-1.** Vicious Cycle of Stigma.

# Evaluating Psychological Fitness and Deployability

The first component of the reintegration function—assessing and making decisions about psychological fitness and deployability—is performed by commanders and other unit leaders by considering four questions:

- Does the Marine or Sailor meet medical standards for retention?
- Is the Marine or Sailor unable to adequately perform required duties because of a stress injury or illness?
- Is the Marine or Sailor unable to adequately perform required duties because of treatment being received for a stress injury or illness?
- Is the Marine or Sailor ineligible for assignment to specific duties because of directives or regulations?

Procedures for answering these questions are described in the next section and summarized in appendix K, *Guidelines for Evaluating Psychological Fitness and Deployability*.

## Evaluating Limitations Due to a Stress Injury or Illness

The crucial first step in the process of reintegrating unit members who have experienced a stress injury or illness—evaluating their current fitness, suitability, and deployability—requires commanders and other leaders to gather information from many different sources from before the onset of the stress injury or illness to the present. They seek input and opinions from all key individuals, including unit medical and religious ministry personnel, treating mental health professionals, family members, peers, and, most importantly, other members of the chain of command. The perceptions and opinions of these sources of information may differ greatly and vary over time, either as the Service member in question recovers from his or her stress injury and regains previous capabilities or as limitations or vulnerabilities come gradually to light during training exercises or operations.

It may be hard to build a consensus view regarding the psychological fitness of a stress-injured Service member because it can be very difficult for others observing that individual to do so objectively, without letting their own biases, preconceptions, and stigmatizing values interfere more than is the case with Marines and Sailors who have been physically injured. Some observers may feel excessively sorry for the psychologically wounded person, while others may feel excessively critical and blaming. Making a decision about fitness and suitability in such cases requires a wise and patient commander or leader who continually evaluates unit members for possible psychological limitations due to stress reactions, injuries, or illnesses. These evaluations should continue throughout deployment cycles and not wait until just before a scheduled deployment.

Appendix K provides an overview of specific sources of information to be consulted and considerations to be made when evaluating possible unit member limitations due to a stress injury or illness. These guidelines for forming judgments and making decisions regarding psychological fitness and deployability are based on the Assistant Secretary of Defense for Health Affairs by policy memorandum of 07 Nov 2006. The office of the Assistant Secretary of Defense for Health Affairs and the Navy Bureau of Medicine and Surgery (BUMED) can provide the most recent updates in policy guidance.

## Evaluating Limitations Due to Psychological Treatments

The most important factors to consider in evaluating psychological fitness, suitability, and deployability are those directly relating to the distress and impairment of normal functioning that may accompany a stress injury or illness. Most Marines and Sailors who meet the criteria for psychological wellness and readiness will be considered "good to go;" however, a second set of criteria to consider in evaluating fitness and deployability are those that relate to the treatments being given by medical and mental health professionals, rather than the symptoms of the stress injuries or illnesses. Psychological treatments can impact fitness for duty and deployment either because the side effects of the treatment, such as with certain medications, may interfere with adequate performance of duties or because sudden withdrawal of the treatment during deployment because it is no longer available may lead to serious worsening of the underlying stress symptoms or to other withdrawal symptoms. Medical and mental health professionals are the primary sources of information in assessing limitations in psychological fitness and deployability due to the side effects of treatment or risks from sudden withdrawal. Appendix K also addresses considerations these professionals might make regarding a Service member who is being treated with psychiatric medication.

## Evaluating Limitations Due to Directives or Other Regulations

The final factor for commanders and leaders to consider while evaluating Marines and Sailors for psychological fitness and suitability is whether any written directives, laws, or other regulations apply to the specific situation under consideration. Such directives are few in number and limited in scope but subject to rapid change, so they will not be directly cited in this publication; however, table 6-1, on page 6-8, cites examples of Department of Defense and Department of the Navy directives that may apply to the evaluation of Service members for fitness, suitability, and deployability.

# Reducing Stigma to Promote Reintegration

The reintegration function of COSC and OSC does not end with the evaluation of psychological fitness, suitability, and deployability. The greatest challenges of reintegration may only begin after a decision is made to return a Marine or Sailor recovering from a stress reaction, injury, or illness to previous duties, to retrain for other duties, or to recommend a medical separation. These challenges are similar to those faced by Service members recovering from physical rather than psychological injuries. In both cases, the reintegration process often involves relearning skills, regaining confidence, and reearning the trust of other team members and shipmates. In the case of recovery from psychological injuries, however, reintegration may be made much more complex and difficult because of the stigma often associated with psychological injuries. For this reason, successful re-integration after a stress injury or illness—whether back to duty or out of the military—depends on winning the battle against stigma.

**Table 6-1.**Regulatons Regarding Psychological Fitness and Suitability.

| Subject | Directives |
|---|---|
| Psychological screening of recruits | DODI 6130.4, *Medical Standards for Appointment, Enlistment, or Induction in the Armed Forces* |
| Suitability screening for overseas or remote duty assignment | OPNAVINST 1300.14, *Suitability Screening for Overseas and Remote Duty Assignment*<br>MCO P1300.8, *Marine Corps Personnel Assignment Policy* |
| Mental health evaluations of members of the armed forces | DODI 6490.1, *Mental Health Evaluations of Members of the Armed Forces*<br>DODI 6490.4, *Requirements for Mental Health Evaluations of Members of the Armed Forces*<br>SECNAVINST 6320.24, *Mental Health Evaluations of Members of the Armed Forces* |
| Personnel security program | DODI 5200.2, *Personnel Security Program*<br>SECNAVINST 5510.30, *Department of the Navy Personnel Security Program* |
| Change to the mental health question (#21) of SF-86, Security Clearance Questionnaire | SecDef Memo of 18 Apr 08, *Policy Implementation—Mental Health Question, Standard Form (SF) 86, Questionnaire for National Security Positions.*<br>CNO Memo of 01 May 08, *Immediate Policy Implementation—Mental Health Question, Standard Form (SF) 86, Questionnaire for National Security Positions.* |
| Navy policies on small arms qualifications while taking psychiatric medications | OPNAVINST 3591.1, *Small Arms Training and Qualification* |
| Physical disability evaluation | DODI 1332.38, *Discharge Review Board (DRB) Procedures and Standards*<br>SECNAVINST 1850.4, *Department of the Navy (DON) Disability Evaluation Manual* |
| Enlisted administrative separations | SECNAVINST 1910.4, *Enlisted Administrative Separations Officer administrative separations* |
| Officer administrative separations | SECNAVINST 1920.6, *Administrative Separations of Officer* |

Legend:

CNO Memo—Chief of Naval Operations memorandum
DODI—Department of Defense instruction
MCO—Marine Corps order
OPNAVINST—Chief of Naval Operations instruction
SecDef Memo—Secretary of Defense memorandum
SECNAVINST—Secretary of the Navy instruction
SF—standard form

The following are examples of stereotypes that can fuel the discrimination of stigma:

- Anyone who experiences overwhelming terror or horror in a life-threatening situation is weak.
- Once a person loses emotional control in a stressful situation, they can never again be trusted to remain tough and steady under pressure.
- Anyone who complains of continued distress or loss of function more than a day or two after a stressful situation is faking.
- Psychiatric medications are crutches rather than real treatments for real health problems.

Labeling such beliefs as stereotypes doesn't mean there are not instances when these beliefs contain elements of truth or that individuals who have been injured by stress do not have limitations and vulnerabilities. What makes them stereotypes and instances of prejudice is the way such beliefs are sometimes applied to situations *before* the facts are known or *instead* of learning the facts. The discrimination of stigma can interfere with reintegration on any of three different levels—organizational, unit, and individual (see table 6-2)—all of which must be addressed by leaders in order to promote successful reintegration.

At the level of the organization—such as the Navy or Marine Corps as a whole—stigma can influence the establishment and continuation of policies that excessively limit the opportunities for service, deployment, or advancement of individuals who have experienced psychological injuries. Organizational policies are based on stigma and prejudice to the extent that they substitute worst case generalizations for case-by-case determinations.

**Table 6-2.** Impact of Stigma and Ways to Defeat It at Three Levels.

|  | Organizational Level | Unit Level | Individual Level |
|---|---|---|---|
| **Stigma Impact** | Policies that limit opportunities based on labels rather than proven abilities. | Ostracizing unit members who are recovering from psychological injuries. | Demoralization and loss of hope. |
| **Ways to Defeat Stigma** | Determine fitness, suitability, and deployability based on performance rather than worst case expectations. | Setting an example of respect and fairness and having zero tolerance for stereotyping in unit. | Education, understanding, and mentorship of those who have successfully recovered from psychological injuries. |

At the level of the unit, stigma can interfere with the mutual trust, respect, and communication that is essential for unit cohesion and the successful reintegration of a stress-impacted unit member. Unit members who hold prejudicial attitudes may be unfairly critical, rejecting, or hostile toward those who have been affected by stress.

At the level of the individual Service member, stigma can takes its greatest toll—by convincing a Marine or Sailor recovering from a stress reaction or injury that he is incapable of returning to his chosen professions or of living a happy, successful life. At the individual level, stigma steals hope.

Leaders in the Navy and Marine Corps have several weapons at their disposal to defeat stigma. At the organizational level, stigma is defeated by establishing policies that give everyone the same chance to succeed, regardless of what has happened in the past, and that ensure that decisions about fitness and suitability are based on proven abilities rather than a medical diagnosis or other label. These policies must also encourage those who could benefit from help to seek it. At the unit level, leaders can defeat stigma by setting examples of respect and fairness for all and by expecting every unit member to live by these same values. At the individual level, stigma can best be defeated by education and understanding, the worst enemies of all forms of prejudice. Leaders who have experienced stress injuries have the most powerful weapon against stigma at their disposal—setting an example of moral courage and recovery. The best hope for reintegration of those who are recovering from stress injuries is the mentorship of those who have successfully recovered.

Preserving the psychological health of Service members and their families is one of the great challenges facing military leaders today. The types of missions modern military organizations are called upon to perform can expose Service members and their spouses and children to intense and prolonged stress. These include counterinsurgency, other irregular forms of warfare, and limitless varieties of humanitarian assistance and disaster relief operations. Since the modern military is an all volunteer force of limited size, Service members and their units must be recycled repeatedly and often. The Nation has come to expect nothing less than a total commitment to the protection and preservation of psychological health of its precious military manpower assets.

Modern psychological and medical science and religious and other spiritual frameworks offer military leaders understanding and tools to help them meet this challenge. Only commanders and the important links in their chains of command, however, can perform the five core functions of COSC and OSC essential for the prevention, identification, and care of adverse stress outcomes across the stress continuum model. Only military leaders can promote Green Zone wellness and return unit members to the Green Zone once they have experienced serious Yellow Zone stress reactions, Orange Zone stress injuries, or Red Zone stress illnesses.

Additional tools for commanders and other military leaders to use in their COSC and OSC functions are included in the appendices of this publication. Among them are overviews of the COSC and OSC challenges of high risk populations, including Service members and individual augmentees possibly at risk for suicide. See appendix L, *Suicide Prevention*, and appendix M, *Individual Augmentation Program Challenges*.

Also included are overviews of two programs that provide direct mental health support for Marine Corps and Navy units in appendix N, *Marine Corps Operational Stress Control and Readiness Program*, and appendix O, *Special Psychiatric Rapid Intervention Teams*. Appendix P, *Humanitarian Assistance and Disaster Relief/Response Challenges*, is a brief overview of the COSC and OSC challenges of these nonwar missions.

The role in COSC and OSC of several specific categories of support personnel are surveyed in appendix Q, *The Role of Religious Ministry Personnel*; appendix R, *The Role of Unit Medical Personnel in Marine Corps Combat and Operational Stress Control*; appendix S, *The Role of Fleet Medical Personnel in Navy Operational Stress Control*; and appendix T, *The Role of Marine Corps Family Readiness Officers*.

Appendix U, *The Marine Operational Stress Training Program*, gives an overview of the Marine Corps deployment cycle COSC workshops for Marines, leaders, and family members. Finally, appendix V, *Navy Caregiver Occupational Stress Control*, presents an overview of programs in the Navy to care for those who provide COSC and OSC support for others in the Navy and Marine Corps.

# Appendix A

# Posttraumatic Stress Disorder Overview

Posttraumatic stress disorder is one of several Red Zone stress illnesses that can arise in the aftermath of combat or other military operational experiences. It can be one of the most chronically disabling stress illnesses, although it usually is much less severe than it is often portrayed to be in movies and other media. Leaders in the military are responsible for knowing the common signs and symptoms of PTSD so they can help recognize it in their unit members. Leaders must also be familiar with the range of treatments known to be effective for PTSD to ensure that unit members receive the best possible care.

## What Is PTSD?

A stress illness, PTSD can arise after a very close brush with death, such as nearly being killed, witnessing someone else's death or the aftermath of death, or taking another person's life. Although their memories of the event will never go away, most people who experience a life-threat develop no more than a Yellow Zone stress reaction or Orange Zone stress injury, from which they usually recover functionally after a few hours, days, or weeks. It can be thought of as an Orange Zone stress injury that doesn't heal and go away over time as expected; instead, it persists and worsens enough to interfere significantly with life functioning or well-being. The disorder can only be diagnosed by a medical or mental health professional and only in persons whose distress or changes in functioning have persisted for at least 30 days after a life-threatening experience and cause significant problems in life.

## What Causes PTSD?

No one knows for sure what causes Orange Zone stress injuries to persist and worsen over time in those individuals who develop PTSD. Many factors are known to increase the risk for PTSD among those exposed to life-threat, such as risk, stress intensity, duration, and how the individual perceives and responds to the stressful event (see fig. A-1 on page A-2), but such risk factors don't "cause" PTSD. They do, however, make it more likely that a person exposed to a life-threat will develop the illness.

## What are the Signs and Symptoms of PTSD?

Some people mistakenly believe that PTSD is a vague and ill-defined disorder that can have almost any signs and symptoms. The core features of PTSD are remarkably consistent over time and from one individual to another. These features include four cardinal symptoms and several associated sets of symptoms. The four cardinal symptoms of PTSD are the following:

- Re-experiencing the life-threatening event repeatedly, often, and in ways that are distressing and interfere with normal functioning, such as—
  - •• *Nightmares*. The individual will often wake up abruptly with heart pounding and intense emotions of anger or fear.
  - •• *Daytime recollections*. Remembrances that intrude on conscious awareness and that are difficult or impossible to brush aside. Sometimes these are also associated with intense physical and emotional activation, as if the event were reoccurring in the present.
  - •• *Environmental triggers*. Reminders of the life-threatening event by similar experiences in the current environment. These include sights, sounds, or smells that stir thoughts, emotions, or actions that are inappropriate for the current situation.

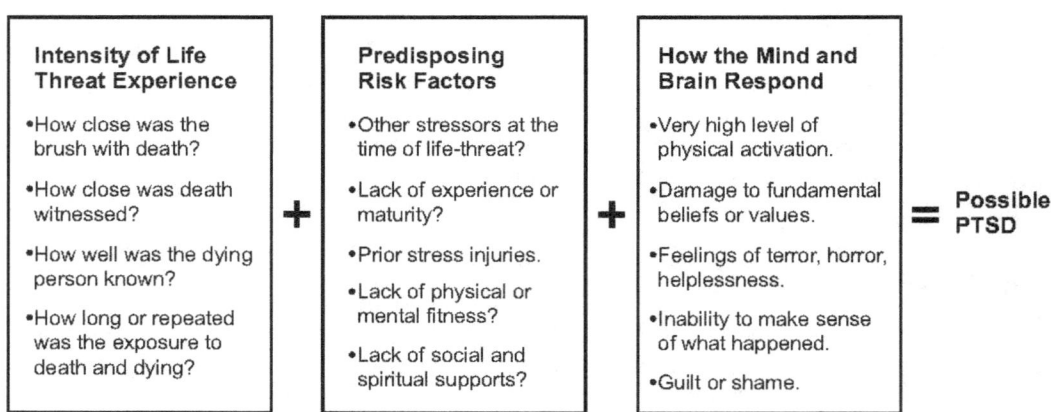

Figure A-1. Interacting Factors That May Lead to Posttraumatic Stress Disorder.

- Numbing of normal emotional responses to nonthreatening life situations, especially those involving intimacy. Close relationships with family and friends suffer and deteriorate.
- Avoiding situations or people that may trigger uncontrollable recollections of the life-threatening experience. The individual spends more time than in the past alone and isolated.
- Excessive physiological activation and emotional intensity that is both uncontrollable and inappropriate for current situations, such as—
  - •• Inability to relax or calm down.
  - •• Difficulty falling or staying asleep.
  - •• Increased and persistent feelings of anger or anxiety.
  - •• Attacks of panic, with pounding heart and rapid breathing.
  - •• Attacks of rage, also with a high degree of physical activation.
  - •• Persistent, intense startle responses to loud noises or other triggers.
  - •• Being constantly "on guard" and scanning for threats even when unnecessary.

These four cardinal symptoms of PTSD are often associated with a number of secondary symptoms, such as the following:

- Alcohol or drug abuse.
- Reckless or thrill-seeking behavior.
- Depression.
- Suicidal or homicidal thoughts or actions.
- Aggressive or violent behavior.

## What are the Best Treatments for PTSD?

Effective treatments for PTSD can be divided into two important and useful categories—treatments that lessen the severity of symptoms or disability but do not actually promote healing of the underlying psychological and biological wounds of PTSD and treatments that actually promote healing. This distinction is an important one, since individuals who receive only treatments that are designed to reduce symptom severity, but no treatments capable of actually promoting healing, may be unlikely to achieve maximum recovery. Table A-1, on page A-4, lists currently available and proven-effective (evidence-based) biological, psychological, social, and spiritual treatments for PTSD.

Table A-1. Types of Treatment for Posttraumatic Stress Disorder.

| Type of Treatment | Lessen Symptoms or Disability | Promote Healing and Recovery |
|---|---|---|
| **Biological** | Sleeping medications, such as Ambien. Tranquilizer medications, such as Ativan, in acute situations. Antidepressant medications, such as Zoloft, if taken at low doses or for less than 12 months. Physical fitness program, including yoga. Healthy diet. Abstinence from alcohol and drugs of abuse, including tobacco. | Antidepressant medications, such as Zoloft, but *only* if taken at high-enough doses and for at least 12 months. |
| **Psychological** | Supportive therapy, such as talking therapy that aims to solve life problems, educate, and encourage, but not to repeatedly and methodically retell life-threat events. Meditation, such as mindfulness meditation or transcendental meditation. | Exposure therapy—repeatedly retelling a distressing story of life-threat to a trained therapist in order to become desensitized to it. Cognitive therapy—repeatedly retelling a story of a life-threat to a trained therapist to discover and change distorted beliefs and ideas about the event, such as exaggerated self-blame. Eye-movement desensitization and reprogramming, a combination of exposure and cognitive therapies. |
| **Social** | Group therapies based on supportive techniques, including problem solving, education, and encouragement. Family or couples therapy. Recreational therapy, such as engaging in sports or hobbies with others recovering from PTSD. | Peer support from others with similar experiences that includes the retelling of stories of a life-threat. Group therapies based on exposure or cognitive processing techniques. |
| **Spiritual** | Religious worship and other practices. Prayer. | Finding meaning and making sense of experiences of a life-threat from spiritual beliefs and activities. |

# Can Marines or Sailors With PTSD Remain on Active Duty?

Yes, they can. A diagnosis of PTSD does not preclude continued service in the military. A medical discharge for PTSD is warranted only if the symptoms that remain after at least 12 months of appropriate and targeted treatment continue to interfere significantly with the performance of required duties.

## How Do the Five COSC and OSC Functions Apply to PTSD Prevention and Treatment?

The five functions apply to PTSD in the following ways:

- *Strengthen.* The first principle of COSC and OSC is to build resilience through tough, realistic training. The current process for training and development of Marine and Navy leaders already provides an excellent framework for building the skills and cohesion necessary. In addition to developing the technical and tactical proficiency of their job, leaders must also build in the skills and habits of good stress management. They can do this by incorporating stress management as part of the training they already do.
- *Mitigate.* Whenever possible, leaders must anticipate and plan for the possibility of severe stressors and ensure that stress levels are well-managed in order to conserve physical, mental, and spiritual health and well-being.
- *Identify.* When severely stressful events occur, leaders need to recognize when their Marines or Sailors are in distress. This recognition can be difficult because most people will tend to minimize or deny that there is a problem. Leaders need to learn to use the COS first aid approach.
- *Treat.* Stress first aid strategies can be effective, but when the Marine or Sailor does not return to normal function, the leader must ensure he or she gets the help needed from the appropriate medical or spiritual professional. The leaders must accept and support the Marine or Sailor being treated for stress injuries as they would other types of injuries.
- *Reintegrate.* The leader must ensure that the Marine or Sailor with a stress injury, who is undergoing or has completed treatment, continues to be an integral part of the unit. The leader's role in supporting the treatment process is to ensure that the Marine or Sailor with a stress injury never becomes a scapegoat or is isolated or shunned because of that injury or because he chose to get help for it. Admitting a need for help and getting it should be seen as a sign of courage and strength.

# APPENDIX B

# TRAUMATIC BRAIN INJURY OVERVIEW

Traumatic brain injury is a physical disruption of neurons in the brain due to a blow to the head or the effects inside the skull of a pressure wave from a nearby blast. It is not known how many Service members deployed to Iraq or Afghanistan have sustained a significant TBI, since many of the milder cases are never reported by the individual. Medical experts also do not yet fully understand the physics and physiology of TBI from blasts, although much research is currently underway. Leaders throughout the Navy and Marine Corps must have a basic understanding of the causes and possible symptoms of TBI so they can identify unit members who may have sustained a brain injury—perhaps even while deployed as an individual augmentee with another unit. Leaders must also know how to manage TBI in their Marines and Sailors so they can properly protect the health and welfare of individuals with TBI and those who depend on them in operational settings. There are three types of physical force that can cause TBI; they can occur separately, simultaneously, or in succession and may be caused by—

- An object striking the head, such as a bullet, fragment, or rock.
- The head striking an object, such as the ground or other hard surface.
- A blast overpressure wave striking the head.

As with Orange Zone stress injuries, TBI damage ranges from the very mild to the very severe. Also similar to stress reactions and injuries, TBI can be cumulative over time, such that even mTBI renders the individual more vulnerable to being damaged by the next physical force to the head.

## How Do Physical Forces Damage the Brain?

There are four major mechanisms by which physical forces impacting the brain can cause damage to nerve cells and the loss of brain function. These four mechanisms, ranging from the most obvious to the most subtle, are described in table B-1 on page B-2.

The first mechanism (penetrating wound) is obvious and unmistakable. The second and third mechanisms (intracranial bleeding and bruising) can develop more slowly and subtly, but are recognizable on standard brain scans, such as an MRI [magnetic resonance imaging] or CT [computed tomography] scan. The fourth mechanism—the mildest and possibly the most common—may not show up on brain scans or any other currently available test, which makes the diagnosis of TBI in its milder forms difficult and controversial.

Table B-1. Four Major Mechanisms that Cause Damage to Nerve Cells.

|  | What It Is | Examples |
|---|---|---|
| **Penetrating Wounds** | One or more objects have pierced the skull and damaged the brain. | Bullet wound to the head. Explosion removes a portion of the skull and brain. Fragments enter the skull. |
| **Intracranial Bleeding** | The skull is not pierced, but blood vessels (arteries or veins) on or in the brain are torn and bleed inside the skull. | Subdural hematoma (blood clot slowly forming under the covering of the brain) from a sharp blow on the head from a fall or explosion. |
| **Intracranial Contusion** | The skull is not pierced and no blood vessels are torn, but the brain is bruised from shifting forcefully inside the skull. | A sharp blow on the head from a fall or explosion causes brief unconsciousness and persistent concussion symptoms. |
| **Stretching of Neurons** | The skull is not pierced, blood vessels are not torn, and the brain is not literally bruised, but the forceful shifting of the brain inside the skull stretches long, thin nerve fibers to the point of injury and possible death. | A sharp blow on the head from a fall or explosion causes brief unconsciousness and concussion symptoms. A blast pressure wave alone (without a blow to the head) causes damage to nerve fibers in the brain and concussion symptoms, sometimes even without loss of consciousness. |

# How is the Severity of TBI Categorized by Medical Personnel?

Aside from the mechanism of injury, TBI is commonly categorized as mild, moderate, or severe based entirely on the degree of disruption in brain function at the time of the injury. Although medical professionals are responsible for diagnosing the severity of a TBI in a Service member, leaders in the Marine Corps and Navy should understand this method of classification so they can communicate with health care providers, make the best possible decisions about fitness for hazardous duty, and ensure that unit members receive the best possible care.

Grading the severity of a TBI and assessing brain function is done in all medical situations through the use of the Glasgow Coma Scale (GCS). The GCS is a simple test, requires no special instruments, can be performed by any trained medical person, and includes only three questions to assess level of consciousness—

- Are the person's eyes open? (scored between 1 and 4).
- Can the person speak? (scored between 1 and 5).
- Can the person move? (scored between 1 and 6).

Each question or item on the GCS is scored according to degree of responsiveness, with higher numbers indicating greater alertness and consciousness and lower numbers indicating deeper degrees of unconsciousness or coma. A perfect score (fully awake and alert) is 15 (4 for eyes spontaneously open, 5 for spontaneous verbal responses, and 6 for movement on command). The lowest possible score is three (one for each item). The GCS score in the aftermath of a head trauma determines the severity of the TBI according to the scoring shown in table B-2.

Table B-2. Glasgow Coma Scale Scoring Chart.

| Lowest GCS Score | TBI severity |
|---|---|
| 3-8 | Severe TBI |
| 9-12 | Moderate TBI |
| 13-15 | mTBI |

Cases of mTBI account for 80 percent of all TBIs in the current theaters of war, while moderate and severe TBI each account for another 10 percent. The most common form of TBI among those deployed to combat zones has been little, if any, observed alteration in consciousness. In cases in which no loss of consciousness was observed, the diagnosis of mTBI requires that the individual experience some other significant change in mental functioning in the immediate aftermath of a head trauma, such as—

• Amnesia—loss of memory after the event.
• Disorientation—loss of accurate awareness of time, date, and location.
• Confusion—difficulty thinking clearly and rationally.

## What are the Later Symptoms of TBI?

Traumatic brain injuries that are moderate or severe are easily recognized because they usually follow a significant period of unconsciousness—30 minutes to 6 hours for moderate TBI and more than 6 hours for severe TBI—and are usually associated with obvious changes in brain function, such as paralysis or loss of sensation. Conversely, mTBI can produce very subtle symptoms that can be difficult to distinguish from the symptoms of a stress injury and can produce no objective evidence of loss of nerve function. Fortunately, the normal course for mTBI is for the symptoms to resolve on their own over a few days or weeks following the event—approximately 90 percent resolve completely. For those in whom mTBI symptoms do not completely resolve, the following are common:

• Blurred vision or eyes tiring easily.
• Persistent headaches or ringing in the ears.
• Trouble with memory, maintaining concentration, or attention.
• Increased sensitivity to lights or sounds.
• Impulsivity or decreased inhibition.
• Persistent lightheadedness or dizziness.
• Slowed thinking, reading, or speaking.
• Emotional irritability or quickness to anger.

# How Should Commanders Manage TBI in Unit Members?

In cases of moderate or severe TBI, the need for ongoing medical care and possible limitations to fitness for duty will be readily apparent. Cases of mTBI, which are far more common in operational units exposed to IEDs and other blast sources, can present more difficult challenges for leaders and caregivers. The following are current Department of Defense guidelines (see *Multi-National Corps-Iraq [MNC-I] Policy on Mild Traumatic Brain Injury*) for leaders and health care professionals for the assessment and management of Service members with possible TBI in a deployed setting (see fig. B-1 on pages B-8 and B-9):

- If TBI is suspected, medical personnel, such as a corpsman or doctor, should perform a thorough evaluation as soon as possible, including a GCS and neurological examination.
- If there is no evidence of moderate to severe TBI or other cause for immediate concern, such as red flags or amber flags as described in fig. B-1, medical personnel should observe the individual perform physical exertion until his heart rate reaches 65 to 85 percent of target heart rate (THR), which equals 220 minus the age of the individual. For example the THR for a 20-year-old would be 200, so exertion testing would continue until the heart rate reached at least 65 to 85 percent of the THR, or 130 to 170 beats per minute.
- If exertion testing produced no TBI symptoms, the individual should then be assessed for more subtle impairment using the Defense and Veterans Brain Injury Center's Military Acute Concussion Evaluation (MACE) tool (available online from http://www.pdhealth.mil/downloads/MACE.pdf).
- If the MACE is in the normal range (scored 25 to 30 out of a possible 30), the individual can be immediately returned to full duty with medical follow-ups as needed.
- If the MACE shows mild impairment (24 or less), the individual should rest for 24 to 48 hours, then the MACE should be repeated.
- If the repeated MACE score remains 24 or less, the individual should be referred to a mental health professional.

## How are the Five Core COSC and OSC Functions Applied to TBI?

Leaders are responsible for ensuring that a basic knowledge and understanding of TBI exists throughout the force. Early detection and intervention results in a better outcome. Battle buddies and fellow shipmates have a similar role in bringing these warning signs to leadership's attention. The five core COSC and OSC functions apply to TBI in the following ways:

- *Strengthen.* The best method of prevention is to avoid all causes of brain injury. In tactical situations, Sailors and Marines should wear Kevlar and load-bearing equipment. In garrison, the consistent use of bicycle/motorcycle helmets and motor vehicle seat belts is required at all times.
- *Mitigate.* If a Sailor or Marine reports having his "bell rung," leaders should listen and watch for subtle changes in behavior or minor complaints or symptoms, which may be signs of mTBI and take actions to conserve physical health and well-being. Leaders should allow a "time out" or a rest period when possible to avoid reinjury until the individual is fully recovered.
- *Identify.* Buddies are a good resource for recognizing subtle changes that may be present if a Sailor or Marine experiences a possible mTBI. Leaders should ensure all Sailors and Marines receive training on the causes and signs of TBI and the importance of early recognition and treatment.
- *Treat.* Every Sailor, Marine, leader, and warfighter should complete a predeployment neurocognitive assessment, referred to as NCAT [Neurocognitive Assessment Tool]. If injury is suspected, performing a MACE is the next step. If a Sailor or Marine reports lightheadedness, dizziness, ringing in the ears, or blurry vision, then time for rest and adequate fluids and food intake should be allowed.
- *Reintegrate.* Postdeployment reintegration is often challenging. Individuals with continued mTBI problems should adhere to consistent and well-structured daily schedules and routines. Writing down notes and reminders may be helpful. Service members should be encouraged to do only one thing at time with minimal distraction. Alcohol should be avoided as it slows healing.

This page intentionally left blank

## Guideline only.
## Not a substitute for clinical judgement.

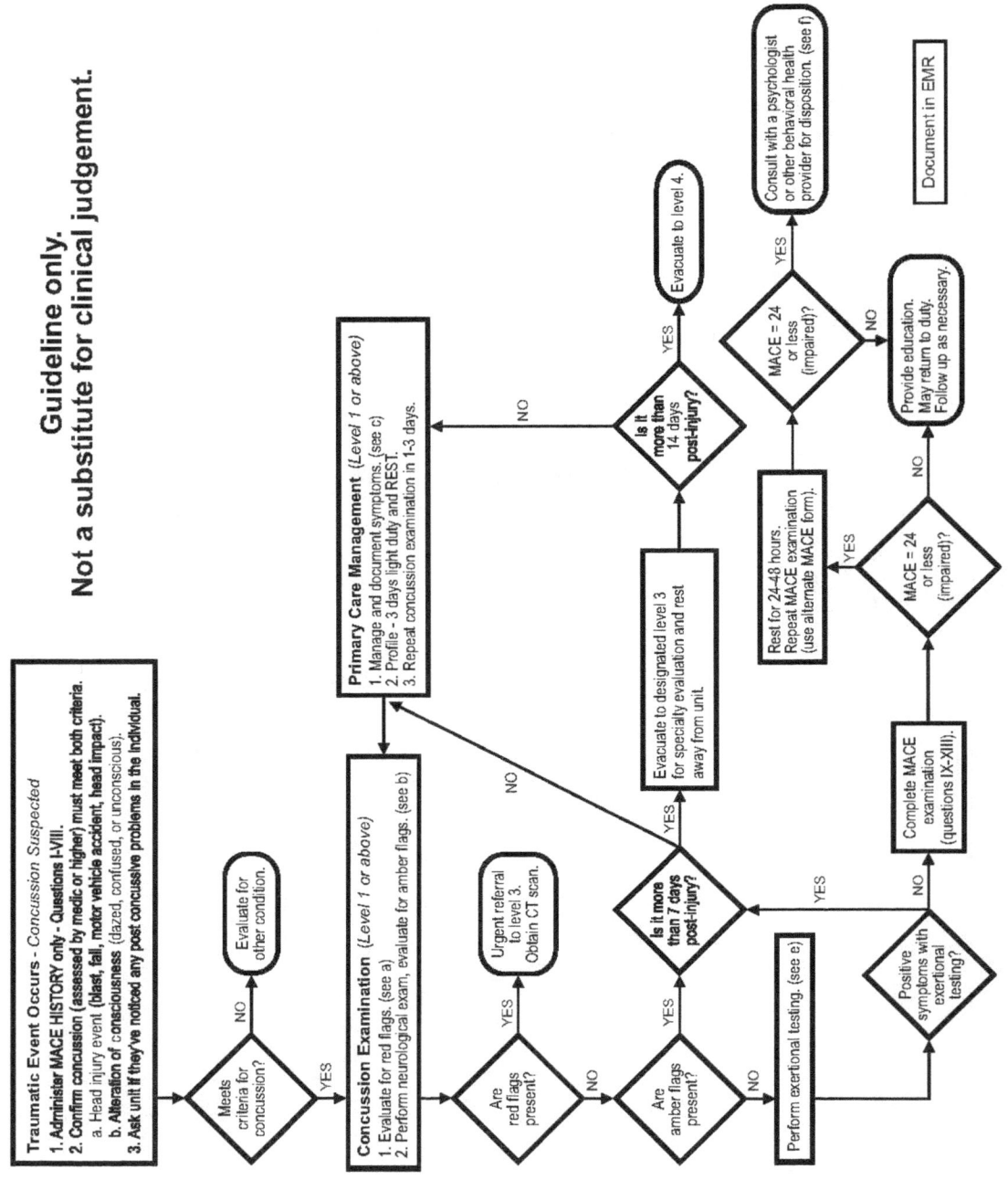

**Traumatic Event Occurs** - *Concussion Suspected*
1. Administer MACE HISTORY only - Questions I-VIII.
2. Confirm concussion (assessed by medic or higher) must meet both criteria.
   a. Head injury event (blast, fall, motor vehicle accident, head impact).
   b. Alteration of consciousness (dazed, confused, or unconscious).
3. Ask unit if they've noticed any post concussive problems in the individual.

Meets criteria for concussion?

NO → Evaluate for other condition.

YES

**Concussion Examination** (*Level 1 or above*)
1. Evaluate for red flags. (see a)
2. Perform neurological exam, evaluate for amber flags. (see b)

Are red flags present?

YES → Urgent referral to level 3. Obtain CT scan.

NO

Are amber flags present?

YES → Evaluate to designated level 3 for specialty evaluation and rest away from unit.

NO

Perform exertional testing. (see e)

Positive symptoms with exertional testing?

YES → Is it more than 7 days post-injury?

NO → Complete MACE examination (questions IX-XIII).

Is it more than 7 days post-injury?

YES → **Primary Care Management** (*Level 1 or above*)
1. Manage and document symptoms. (see c)
2. Profile - 3 days light duty and REST.
3. Repeat concussion examination in 1-3 days.

NO →

**Primary Care Management** (*Level 1 or above*)

Is it more than 14 days post-injury?

YES → Evaluate to level 4.

NO →

MACE = 24 or less (impaired)?

YES → Rest for 24-48 hours. Repeat MACE examination (use alternate MACE form).

NO → Provide education. May return to duty. Follow up as necessary.

MACE = 24 or less (impaired)?

YES → Consult with a psychologist or other behavioral health provider for disposition. (see f)

NO → Provide education. May return to duty. Follow up as necessary.

Document in EMR

**B-8** MCRP 6-11C/NTTP 1-15M Combat and Operational Stress Control

## Legend

| | |
|---|---|
| EMR | electronic medical record |
| ICD | International Classification of Diseases |
| LOC | loss of consciousness |
| NSAID | nonsteroidal anti-inflammatory drug |
| THR | target heart rate |

### (a) Red Flags:

1. Progressively declining level of consciousness.
2. Progressive declining neurological exam.
3. Pupillary asymmetry.
4. Seizures.
5. Repeated vomiting.
6. Clinician verified GCS<15.
7. LOC>5 minutes.
8. Double vision.
9. Worsening headache.
10. Neurological deficit: motor or sensory.
11. Cannot recognize people or disoriented to place.
12. Neurological ataxia.

### (b) Amber Flags (persisting beyond initial traumatic event):

1. Confusion.
2. Slurred speech.
3. Unusual behavior.
4. Unsteady on feet.
5. Weakness.
6. Vertigo/dizziness.
7. Headache.

### (c) Primary Care Management:

1. Give educational sheet to all MBTI patients.
2. Headache management - use acetaminophen.
3. Avoid tramadol, narcotics, NSAIDs, aspirin, or other platelet inhibitors until cleared for return to duty.
4. Consider neurology referral or evacuate to higher level if clinically indicated.
5. Screen for anxiety and depression.
6. Document concussion diagnosis in EMR. (see d)

### (d) ICD-9 Codes:

850.0   Concussion without LOC.
850.11 Concussion with LOC≤30 min.
850.12 Concussion with LOC 31-59 min.
E979.2 Injury from terrorist explosion blast.

### (e) Exertional Testing Protocol:

1. 65-85% THR (THR = 220-age) using push-up, step aerobic, treadmill, hand crank.
2. Assess for symptoms (headache, vertigo, photophobia, balance, dizziness, nausea, tinnitus, visual changes, response to bright light or loud noise).

### (f) Psychology Consult:

1. If a psychologist or other provider can conduct neurocognitive testing at the current location, refer the patient for testing.
2. If no neurocognitive test available at current location, contact the nearest psychologist to discuss the best option. Subsequently, the psychologist in conjunction with the provider and patient's command will weigh the costs and benefits of transporting the patient for further testing versus further rest in place.

# APPENDIX C

# CHECKLIST FOR EVALUATING RESILIENCE IMPACT OF TRAINING

| | |
|---|---|
| ☐ | Is the training realistic and relevant? |
| | ☐ Will the training allow unit members to master the same specific challenges they will probably face during deployment? |
| | ☐ Will the training occur in an environment that mimics the sights, sounds, and smells they will experience during deployment? |
| | ☐ Will the training prepare unit members so thoroughly that there will be few surprises during deployment? |
| ☐ | Will the training encourage unit members to develop new skills and competencies? |
| | ☐ Will the training push unit members beyond their current level of knowledge and skill? |
| | ☐ Will the increase in knowledge and skill continue during training? |
| ☐ | Will the training provide experiences of success and mastery? |
| | ☐ Will the training set expectations that will be tough but achievable? |
| | ☐ Will unit members be able to keep trying until they master each challenge? |
| ☐ | Will the training encourage unit members to solve problems in unfamiliar situations? |
| | ☐ Does the training include opportunities to think, plan, and decide, as well as to respond to known situations with rehearsed patterns of action? |
| | ☐ Will the training encourage team problem solving? |
| ☐ | Will the training inoculate unit members to likely intense operational stressors? |
| | ☐ If unit members may face life-threat during deployment, does training mimic life-threat in a subdued, tolerable form? |
| | ☐ If unit members may face the aftermath of violence during deployment, does training include exposure to the sights, sounds, and smells of death or injury? |
| | ☐ Does the training include a mechanism for leaders to monitor unit members' responses to stress to ensure they react with progressively less alarm? |
| ☐ | Do safeguards exist to prevent stress injuries during training? |
| | ☐ Will leaders continuously monitor the stress zones of unit members? |
| | ☐ Will leaders ensure adequate sleep and recovery time? |

| | | |
|---|---|---|
| ☐ | Will the training require unit members to communicate with and trust in each other? | |
| | ☐ | Will the training require and promote teamwork? |
| | ☐ | Will success during training be perceived as team achievements? |
| | ☐ | Does the training include shared hardships and adversities? |
| ☐ | Will the training enhance unit members' communication and trust in unit leaders? | |
| | ☐ | Will the training require vertical communication in the chain of command? |
| | ☐ | Will the training include hardships shared by leaders as well as unit members? |
| | ☐ | Will the training challenge while ensuring the successes of leaders of small units? |
| ☐ | Will the training reinforce core values and ethical decisionmaking? | |
| | ☐ | Will the training include challenges for ethical decisionmaking under stress? |
| | ☐ | Will there be discussions of how core values are reflected in the training? |
| ☐ | Will the training teach stress management and stress first aid knowledge and skills? | |
| | ☐ | Will the training teach self-care and buddy care to reduce and mitigate stress? |
| | ☐ | Will recognition of the stress zones of the stress continuum model be taught? |
| | ☐ | Will the training reduce the stigma attached to getting help for stress injuries? |

# APPENDIX D

# CHECKLIST FOR PRESERVING RESOURCES TO MITIGATE STRESS

| | Resource Category | Stressors to Attack | How to Attack These Stressors | How to Replenish This Resource |
|---|---|---|---|---|
| **PHYSICAL** | **Health and Well-being** | ☐ Sleep deprivation<br>☐ Overexposure to harsh weather<br>☐ Injuries<br>☐ Illnesses | ☐ Sleep discipline<br>☐ Protective equipment<br>☐ Safety precautions<br>☐ Monitor health and well-being | ☐ Rest and down time<br>☐ Physical fitness<br>☐ Training in hygiene and self-care<br>☐ Attend to quality of life everywhere |
| | **Personal Space and Possessions** | ☐ Loss of income<br>☐ Family breakups<br>☐ Loss of personal space | ☐ Help Service members/family members plan for losses of income<br>☐ Inform Service members about deployment schedule<br>☐ Protect personal possessions and space | ☐ Support families throughout deployments<br>☐ Allow time and communication with family<br>☐ Allow time for moonlighting, if warranted |
| **MENTAL and EMOTIONAL** | **Safety and Security** | ☐ Life-threat situations<br>☐ Handling bodies and body parts<br>☐ Unexpected attacks, such as IEDs<br>☐ Being in passive or helpless positions | ☐ Minimize number of close-up experiences of death<br>☐ Hold AARs to restore confidence<br>☐ Prepare for the unexpected<br>☐ Enhance physical safety and security | ☐ Model courage during life-threat<br>☐ Maintain unit cohesion as a fear antidote<br>☐ Train and retrain to increase confidence<br>☐ Keep Service members and family members active, not passive |
| | **Morale** | ☐ Prolonged or repeated deployments<br>☐ Abusive or inconsistent leadership<br>☐ Boredom, lack of accomplishment<br>☐ Not enough information getting to service members | ☐ Get Service members home as soon as possible<br>☐ Be honest about schedule changes<br>☐ Listen to Marines, Sailors, and family members<br>☐ Set and achieve realistic goals continuously | ☐ Vary routines and assignments<br>☐ Rejuvenating unit activities<br>☐ Explain meaning and value of mission<br>☐ Reward accomplishments |
| | **Pride and Self-Esteem** | ☐ Failures or mistakes<br>☐ Excessive self-blame, such as guilt<br>☐ Scapegoating or social shunning | ☐ Mentor correction of mistakes with honor<br>☐ Anticipate and limit self-blame<br>☐ Mentor outliers fully into or out of unit | ☐ Reward individual and unit achievements<br>☐ Share praise and blame appropriately<br>☐ Match responsibilities to abilities |

| | Resource Category | Stressors to Attack | How to Attack These Stressors | How to Replenish This Resource |
|---|---|---|---|---|
| **SOCIAL** | **Peer Support** | □ Unit members joining late or leaving early<br><br>□ Leadership turnover<br><br>□ Ethical violations by unit members<br><br>□ Hazing by peers or abuse by leaders | □ Keep unit members who transfer out part of unit<br><br>□ Ensure leadership continuity<br><br>□ Enforce ethics and law of war<br><br>□ Zero tolerance for hazing or abuse | □ Vertical and horizontal communication<br><br>□ Consistency of leadership<br><br>□ Shared adversity and sacrifices<br><br>□ Shared achievements and victories |
| | **Family Support** | □ Irresolvable family conflicts<br><br>□ Family or relationship breakups<br><br>□ Injuries or illnesses in family members | □ Solve family member problems before deployments<br><br>□ Teach coping and communication skills<br><br>□ Train family members to recognize stress injuries | □ Treat family members like important parts of unit<br><br>□ Support families throughout deployments<br><br>□ Keep communication lines open |
| **SPIRITUAL** | **Meaning and Trust in Values** | □ Ethical violations that go unaddressed<br><br>□ Not adequately honoring the fallen<br><br>□ Events that violate logical expectations<br><br>□ Leaders failing to correct their own mistakes | □ Teach and model moral courage<br><br>□ Live by core values<br><br>□ Memorials and ceremonies to honor dead<br><br>□ AARs to restore meaning | □ Vertical and horizontal communication<br><br>□ Include ethics in all training<br><br>□ Ensure commitment goes both ways<br><br>□ Keep core values in sight |
| | **Faith** | □ Events that contradict beliefs<br><br>□ Betrayals of trust by leaders or peers<br><br>□ Moral dilemmas | □ Restore trust and belief in "goodness"<br><br>□ Model compassion and forgiveness<br><br>□ Mentor resolution of moral dilemmas | □ Encourage spirituality and religion in unit<br><br>□ Model faith and spirituality<br><br>□ Encourage tolerance for faith diversity |

# APPENDIX E

# THE AFTER ACTION REVIEW

The AAR is a traditional method for leaders to gather and share information in a unit after any operational or training event. They discuss correct and incorrect actions and why events proceeded as they did. The primary purpose for AARs is to disseminate lessons learned to improve performance, but they can also serve in operational units as a tool for leaders to perform the five core functions of COSC or OSC—strengthen, mitigate, identify, treat, and reintegrate.

## Key Features of AARs for COSC and OSC

The COSC and OSC AARs are conducted after any event of unusual stress, particularly those involving life-threat, loss of life, serious injury, or potential violations of rules or values. To contribute to the core functions of COSC and OSC, AARs must have the key features of safety, honesty, and meaning:

- *Safety* during AARs must include physical, emotional, or moral safety. Physical safety is assured by conducting AARs in protected locations of low risk for physical harm. Emotional and moral safety are assured by excluding all forms of criticism, reprimand, or investigation for possible censure from AARs and by ensuring that no unit member is forced to divulge their personal reactions to a stressful event if they choose not to.
- *Honesty* is assured by the leader modeling truthful, open, and direct communication and making clear to other unit members that they are expected to do the same. Everyone must be free to speak openly.
- *Meaning* is assured during AARs by developing a common understanding among unit members about why a stressful event occurred and how the actions of the unit contributed to the unit's mission. The AARs should not be concluded until all unit members have made sense out of the events they experienced.

# Procedures for Conducting an After Action Review

The following procedures answer questions regarding who should be involved in an AAR; some of the characteristics of an AAR; and when, where, and how AARs should be conducted.

## Who
- All members of a small unit, such as a squad, fire team, work center, or other small team, who took part in the recent event to be reviewed.
- Members of a staff or chain of command at equivalent level, such as all department heads or all senior staff NCOs, who were directly involved in the recent event to be reviewed.
- A designated facilitator or leader of the AAR, such as the senior leader present.
- No outsiders—only those who are known to unit members and are directly involved in the event to be reviewed.

## What
- A private, uninterrupted meeting in a secure location soon after the event.
- If possible, unit members should be seated facing each other, such as in a circle, rather than being seated in a classroom style in which everyone faces the same direction.

## When
- As soon as practical after an event involving a life-threat, loss of life, serious injury, or potential violations of rules or values, but not before unit members have been rested and replenished.
- Generally, 8 to 48 hours after an unusually stressful event.
- During a "safety stand-down" or operational pause to ensure time to complete the AAR.
- Should be expected to last from 15 to 90 minutes or more.

## Where
- In a safe, secure, and comfortable location where interruptions are unlikely.
- May be conducted indoors or out, in the field or on deck, or in a building or interior space.

## How

- Assemble unit members in the designated AAR location.
- Explain the purpose and rules of the AAR, especially the key features of safety, honesty, and meaning.
- The leader recounts the facts of the recent event to the best of his recollection and understanding.
- Unit members are then encouraged to each recount the facts of the event from their points of view and recollections.
- Differences in perceptions and memories are reconciled, as much as possible, to develop a logical, coherent story of what happened.
- Either during or after this recounting of facts, the leader also communicates significant internal experiences and reactions to the event, such as meaningful or troubling thoughts, feelings, or physical changes.
- Other unit members are encouraged and made to feel safe while sharing their own personal reactions to the event.
- The leader listens and watches for evidence of excessive and unwarranted blame toward self, peers, or leaders, and attempts to neutralize excessive blame through an honest appraisal of the causes for whatever went wrong and an appropriate sharing of the blame.
- The leader gives meaning to the unit's experience by reinforcing what was good, proper, and heroic in unit members' actions and underscoring the ways in which this event contributed to the unit's mission and training. If mistakes were made, the leader states how these mistakes will be avoided in the future.
- All leaders in the unit should watch and listen for unusual distress or changes in functioning among unit members that might be signals of severe Yellow or Orange Zone stress.
- Use the seven Cs of stress first aid to promote recovery and healing as indicated.

## Why

- Strengthen unit members by enhancing their confidence in themselves and their peers, leaders, and equipment and by preparing them to better master similar challenges in the future.
- Mitigate stress in the unit by enhancing unit cohesion, increasing understanding of events, and reducing the potentially toxic impact of negative emotions, such as guilt, shame, and blame.

- Identify stress zones in unit members by watching and listening for severe distress or alterations in normal functioning.
- Treat identified Yellow, Orange, or Red Zone stress, both during and after the AAR, using the seven principals of stress first aid, including referring those who need it for further professional care.
- Reintegrate unit members who feel alienated from their peers because of guilt, shame, or blame and restore mutual trust and respect in the unit.

# APPENDIX F

# ORANGE ZONE BEHAVIOR WARNING SIGNS

| | | NOT AT ALL TRUE | SOMEWHAT TRUE | EXTREMELY TRUE |
|---|---|:---:|:---:|:---:|
| 1 | For a period of time, the individual did not act like his or her normal self. | O | O | O |
| 2 | For a period of time, the individual seemed to feel fearless and invulnerable, as if nothing could harm him or her. | O | O | O |
| 3 | For a period of time, the individual seemed not to care about his or her own or others' welfare or safety. | O | O | O |
| 4 | For a period of time, the individual seemed to feel no remorse for doing things that would have bothered him or her in the past. | O | O | O |
| 5 | For a period of time, the individual seemed to be determined to get revenge. | O | O | O |
| 6 | For a period of time, the individual seemed unable to stop laughing, crying, or screaming. | O | O | O |
| 7 | For a period of time, the individual seemed helpless and unable to look out for his or her own welfare. | O | O | O |
| 8 | For a period of time, the individual appeared to be confused, as if having difficulty making sense of what was happening. | O | O | O |
| 9 | For a period of time, the individual appeared to be disoriented, as if uncertain about where he or she was or what day or time it was. | O | O | O |
| 10 | For a period of time, the individual could not move parts of his or her body. | O | O | O |
| 11 | For a period of time, the individual froze or appeared to be moving very slowly, such that he or she could not do everything desired. | O | O | O |
| 12 | For a period of time, the individual's speech changed, such as stuttering, repeating words or phrases, or having a shaky or squeaky voice. | O | O | O |
| 13 | For a period of time, the individual was not able to fully carry out his or her duties during or immediately after the event. | O | O | O |
| 14 | For a period of time, the individual expressed the belief that he or she was going to die. | O | O | O |
| 15 | For a period of time, the individual had an intense physical reaction, such as sweating, shaking, or heart pounding. | O | O | O |

# APPENDIX G

# STRESS CONTINUUM DECISION FLOWCHART FOR MARINES AND SAILORS

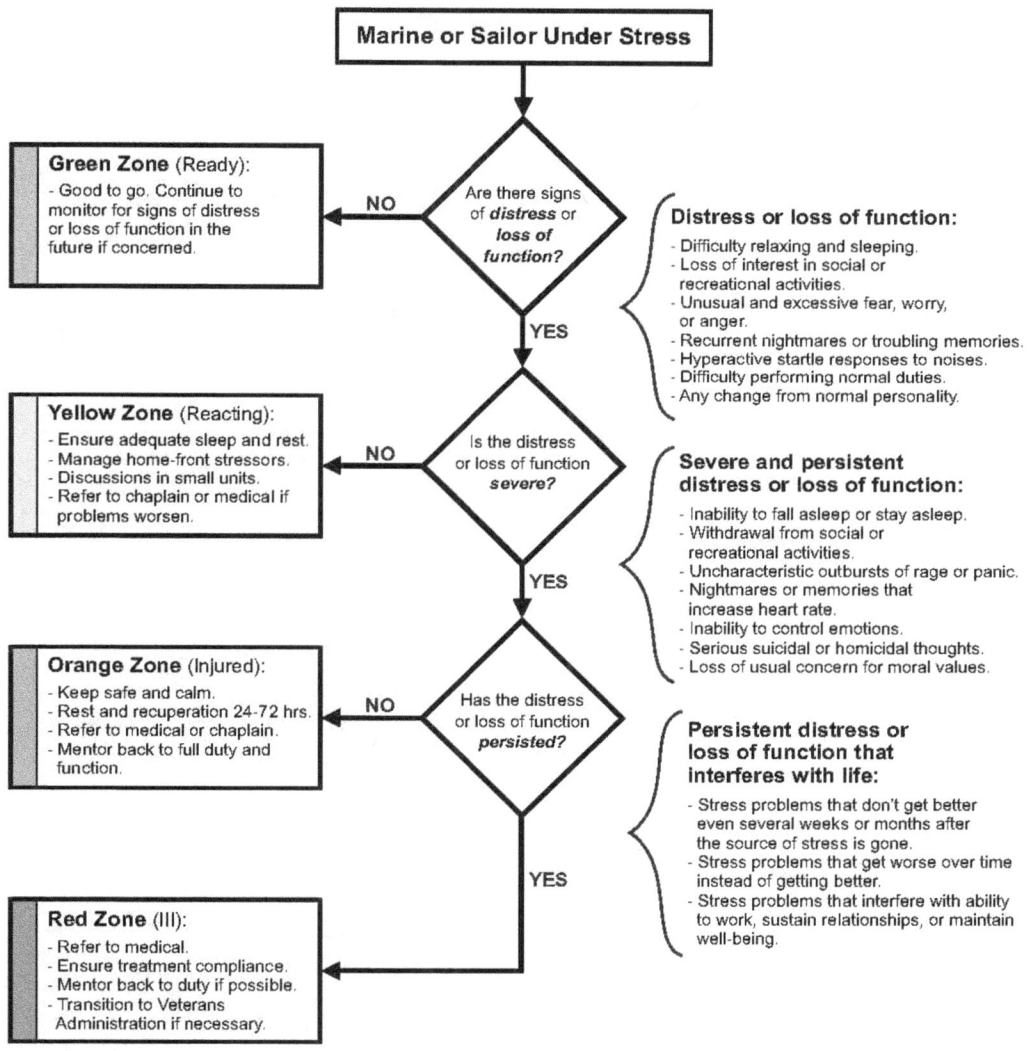

**Marine or Sailor Under Stress**

**Green Zone** (Ready):
- Good to go. Continue to monitor for signs of distress or loss of function in the future if concerned.

**NO** — Are there signs of *distress* or *loss of function?*

**Distress or loss of function:**
- Difficulty relaxing and sleeping.
- Loss of interest in social or recreational activities.
- Unusual and excessive fear, worry, or anger.
- Recurrent nightmares or troubling memories.
- Hyperactive startle responses to noises.
- Difficulty performing normal duties.
- Any change from normal personality.

**YES**

**Yellow Zone** (Reacting):
- Ensure adequate sleep and rest.
- Manage home-front stressors.
- Discussions in small units.
- Refer to chaplain or medical if problems worsen.

**NO** — Is the distress or loss of function *severe?*

**Severe and persistent distress or loss of function:**
- Inability to fall asleep or stay asleep.
- Withdrawal from social or recreational activities.
- Uncharacteristic outbursts of rage or panic.
- Nightmares or memories that increase heart rate.
- Inability to control emotions.
- Serious suicidal or homicidal thoughts.
- Loss of usual concern for moral values.

**YES**

**Orange Zone** (Injured):
- Keep safe and calm.
- Rest and recuperation 24-72 hrs.
- Refer to medical or chaplain.
- Mentor back to full duty and function.

**NO** — Has the distress or loss of function *persisted?*

**Persistent distress or loss of function that interferes with life:**
- Stress problems that don't get better even several weeks or months after the source of stress is gone.
- Stress problems that get worse over time instead of getting better.
- Stress problems that interfere with ability to work, sustain relationships, or maintain well-being.

**YES**

**Red Zone** (Ill):
- Refer to medical.
- Ensure treatment compliance.
- Mentor back to duty if possible.
- Transition to Veterans Administration if necessary.

# STRESS CONTINUUM
# DECISION FLOWCHART FOR SPOUSES

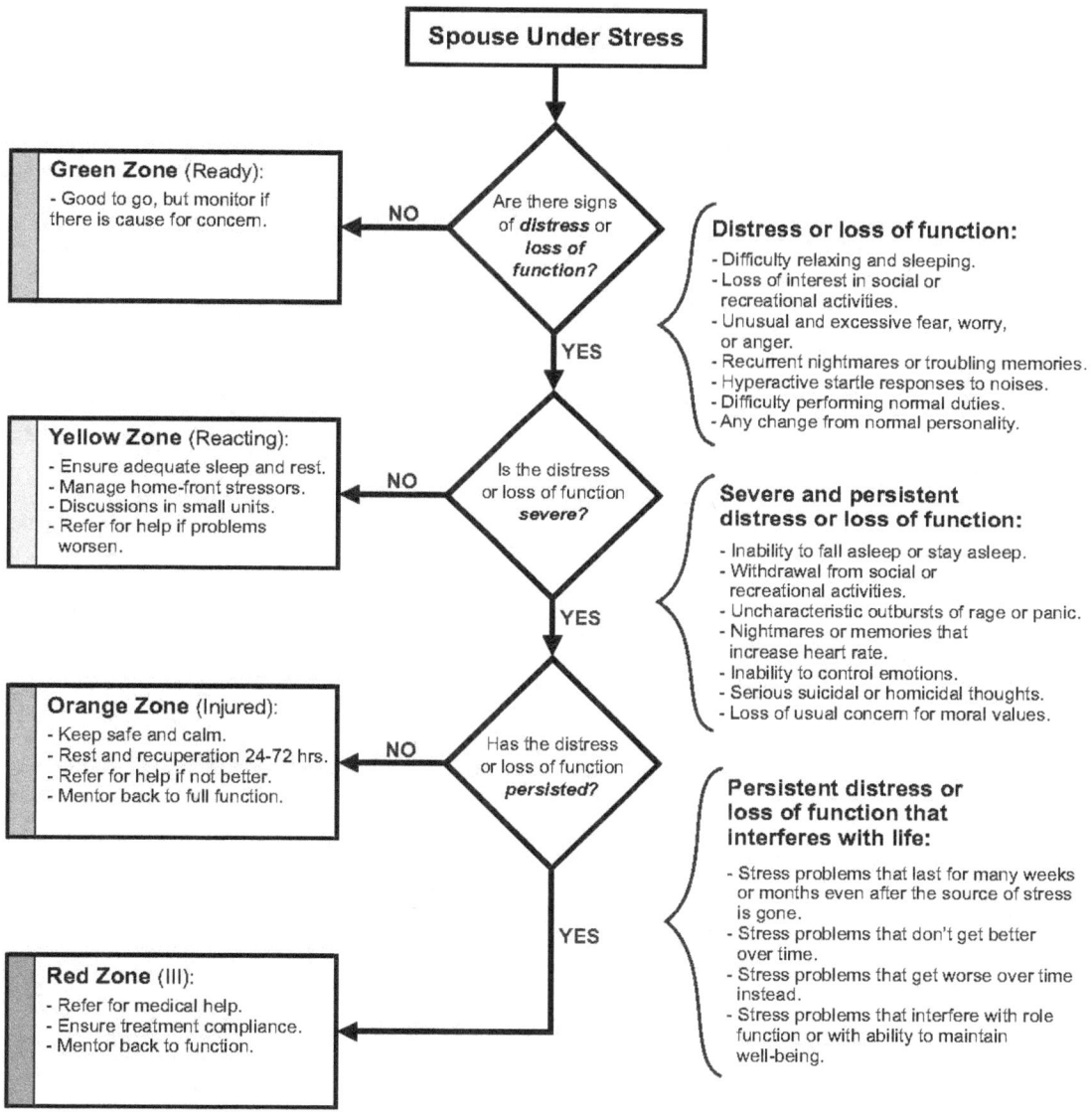

**Spouse Under Stress**

Are there signs of *distress* or *loss of function?*

**Green Zone** (Ready):
- Good to go, but monitor if there is cause for concern.

**NO** →

**YES** ↓

**Distress or loss of function:**
- Difficulty relaxing and sleeping.
- Loss of interest in social or recreational activities.
- Unusual and excessive fear, worry, or anger.
- Recurrent nightmares or troubling memories.
- Hyperactive startle responses to noises.
- Difficulty performing normal duties.
- Any change from normal personality.

Is the distress or loss of function *severe?*

**Yellow Zone** (Reacting):
- Ensure adequate sleep and rest.
- Manage home-front stressors.
- Discussions in small units.
- Refer for help if problems worsen.

**NO** →

**YES** ↓

**Severe and persistent distress or loss of function:**
- Inability to fall asleep or stay asleep.
- Withdrawal from social or recreational activities.
- Uncharacteristic outbursts of rage or panic.
- Nightmares or memories that increase heart rate.
- Inability to control emotions.
- Serious suicidal or homicidal thoughts.
- Loss of usual concern for moral values.

Has the distress or loss of function *persisted?*

**Orange Zone** (Injured):
- Keep safe and calm.
- Rest and recuperation 24-72 hrs.
- Refer for help if not better.
- Mentor back to full function.

**NO** →

**YES** ↓

**Persistent distress or loss of function that interferes with life:**
- Stress problems that last for many weeks or months even after the source of stress is gone.
- Stress problems that don't get better over time.
- Stress problems that get worse over time instead.
- Stress problems that interfere with role function or with ability to maintain well-being.

**Red Zone** (III):
- Refer for medical help.
- Ensure treatment compliance.
- Mentor back to function.

# STRESS CONTINUUM
# DECISION FLOWCHART FOR CHILDREN

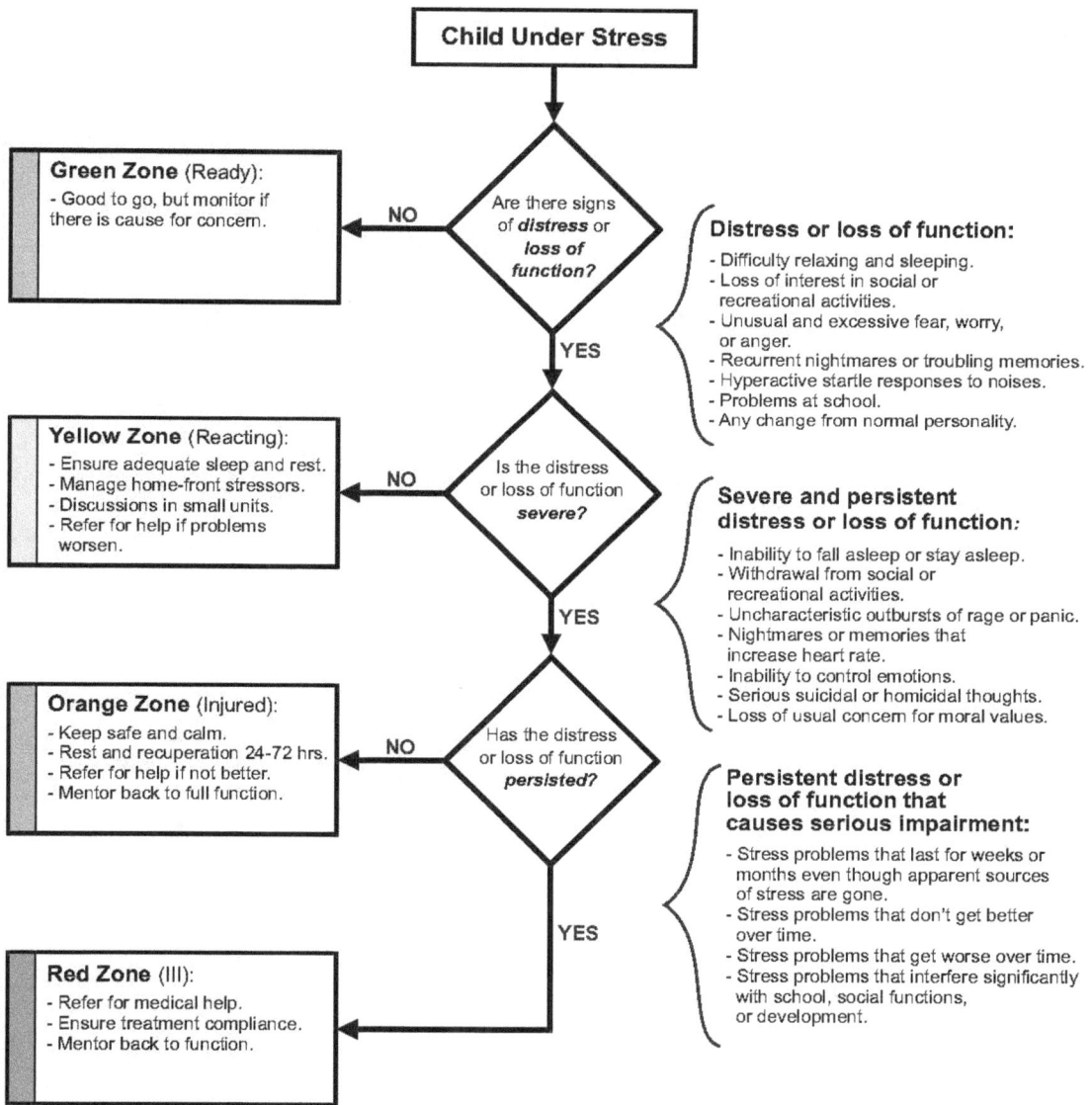

**Child Under Stress**

**Green Zone** (Ready):
- Good to go, but monitor if there is cause for concern.

NO ← Are there signs of *distress* or *loss of function?*

**Distress or loss of function:**
- Difficulty relaxing and sleeping.
- Loss of interest in social or recreational activities.
- Unusual and excessive fear, worry, or anger.
- Recurrent nightmares or troubling memories.
- Hyperactive startle responses to noises.
- Problems at school.
- Any change from normal personality.

YES

**Yellow Zone** (Reacting):
- Ensure adequate sleep and rest.
- Manage home-front stressors.
- Discussions in small units.
- Refer for help if problems worsen.

NO ← Is the distress or loss of function *severe?*

**Severe and persistent distress or loss of function:**
- Inability to fall asleep or stay asleep.
- Withdrawal from social or recreational activities.
- Uncharacteristic outbursts of rage or panic.
- Nightmares or memories that increase heart rate.
- Inability to control emotions.
- Serious suicidal or homicidal thoughts.
- Loss of usual concern for moral values.

YES

**Orange Zone** (Injured):
- Keep safe and calm.
- Rest and recuperation 24-72 hrs.
- Refer for help if not better.
- Mentor back to full function.

NO ← Has the distress or loss of function *persisted?*

**Persistent distress or loss of function that causes serious impairment:**
- Stress problems that last for weeks or months even though apparent sources of stress are gone.
- Stress problems that don't get better over time.
- Stress problems that get worse over time.
- Stress problems that interfere significantly with school, social functions, or development.

YES

**Red Zone** (Ill):
- Refer for medical help.
- Ensure treatment compliance.
- Mentor back to function.

# APPENDIX J

# CALMING AND FOCUSING TECHNIQUES

Military training and operations can be very intense and may stir up strong feelings that may detract from the ability to focus on duties. Letting yourself experience strong feelings at the right time is good, such as when it is safe and you are with people you trust. At other times, however, you may need to maintain control over your emotions and thinking in order to focus on the task at hand. The following strategies can be used when you need to calm yourself down, put your feelings aside, and restore your mental focus.

This appendix offers step-by-step instructions in the practice of two commonly used and effective procedures for calming—deep breathing and grounding. Both can be performed by an individual experiencing excessive levels of physical or emotional activation, either by himself or while being coached by someone else who has recognized the need for calming and is rendering stress first aid. All members of the military, including family members, should become very comfortable and confident in the use of these two procedures. Like safety procedures, they cannot be learned at the time they are really needed. They must be practiced repeatedly in advance so they will happen almost automatically when the need arises.

## Deep Breathing

Taking control of your breathing is a good way to calm yourself down and restore your focus. This is one reason that breathing is stressed in martial arts; it creates a body-mind connection. This connection can help you control how well your body receives oxygen, reduces stress, and increases your self-awareness. Once you get your mind and body in tune with one another, you'll be able to better control your breathing. By controlling your breathing, you'll gain better control over your body, including its emotional reactions. The following actions are techniques to help gain control over breathing:

- Prepare:
  - •• Pause whatever activity you are engaged in, if possible.
  - •• To the extent possible, put yourself in a safe and comfortable position.
  - •• Close your eyes, if you can do so safely.
  - •• Turn your attention to your breath. If other thoughts come to your mind, don't fight them. Just notice that they are there and return your attention to your breath.
- Do:
  - •• Inhale slowly and deeply into the bottom of your lungs, so that your belly rises with the breath.
  - •• Breathe in for a count of 4, hold it for a count of 2, and exhale slowly for the count of 4.
  - •• Let tension leave your body each time you exhale.
- Check and repeat:
  - •• Repeat for 5 to 10 minutes.
  - •• Check in with yourself; if you are still feeling keyed up, repeat the deep breathing until you are feeling calmer and more relaxed.

# Grounding

Grounding is a technique to quickly refocus your thinking if it becomes scattered or fuzzy because of overwhelming stress and intense feelings of fear or anger. It can be used along with deep breathing to produce both relative calmness and more focused thinking. The following actions are grounding techniques:

- Prepare:
  - •• Pause whatever activity you are engaged in, if possible.
  - •• To the extent possible, put yourself in a safe place and comfortable position.
  - •• Keep your eyes open as you prepare to turn your attention from your inner world of distress to the calmer outside world.
- Do:
  - •• Look around you and see that you are safe—there are no immediate threats to your life or safety.
  - •• Notice that the thoughts and feelings you have had that have made you feel unsafe do not belong where you are now.

- •• Try to imagine putting a barrier between you and all of your unsafe feelings by wadding them up, stuffing them into a container, and sealing it.
- •• Imagine the container of your unsafe feelings has been placed behind a thick concrete barricade far away from you.
- •• Look around the place where you are and name as many objects and colors as you can, one by one.
- •• Notice and name what is in front of you, to your left, to your right, behind you, above you, and beneath you.
- •• If you see any printed words, read them and then name each letter backward.
- •• Focus your thoughts on naming things in which you are interested, such as sports teams, types of dogs, the names of entertainers or athletes, or television shows.
- •• Count slowly forward (1 to 10) or backward (10 to 1).
- •• Notice the pressure of your body on the ground or floor.
- •• Stretch and take a deep breath.
- Check and repeat:
  - •• Check in with yourself. If you are still feeling unsafe or your thoughts are unclear and unfocused, repeat these exercises.

# APPENDIX K

# GUIDELINES FOR EVALUATING PSYCHOLOGICAL FITNESS AND DEPLOYABILITY

| Source of Information | | Medical and Mental Health Personnel | Chain of Command and Chaplains |
|---|---|---|---|
| **Service Member is Psychologically Fit and Deployable if:** | **In Spite of a Stress Injury or Illness:** | ☐ Service member meets medical standards for retention.<br>☐ Service member is currently <u>not significantly impaired</u> in performance of duties due to stress injury or illness symptoms.<br>☐ The expected demands of future deployments are <u>not</u> likely to cause Service member to become significantly impaired.<br>☐ Service member is motivated to remain on active duty and deploy.<br>☐ Medical personnel clear Service member for deployment.<br>☐ Medical board for possible disability discharge is warranted.<br>☐ Service member does not require treatment that may be unavailable or impractical during deployment. | ☐ Service member has demonstrated <u>competency</u> in all essential knowledge, skills, and attitudes throughout recent training.<br>☐ Service member is <u>confident</u> in his or her own abilities, in leaders, peers, and equipment.<br>☐ If Service member is not now fully competent or confident, these can be regained in near future.<br>☐ Service member is trusted by other members of the team.<br>☐ Service member contributes positively to cohesion and morale.<br>☐ Service member displays adequate leadership skills.<br>☐ Service member is motivated to remain on active duty and deploy.<br>☐ Chain of command trusts Service member. |
| | **In Spite of Mental Health Treatment:** | ☐ Needed psychotherapy treatment will be concluded within 6 to 12 months.<br>☐ Current medications do <u>not</u> cause potentially impairing side effects.<br>☐ Current medications are on a stable dosage (Service member has been taking the same medication at the same dose for at least 3 months).<br>☐ Medication is safe to take on deployment.<br>☐ No risk for serious withdrawal symptoms if medication is stopped.<br>☐ No risk for serious worsening of symptoms if treatment is stopped. | ☐ Service member is compliant with all prescribed treatments.<br>☐ Chain of command clears Service member to take prescribed medications during deployment. |

**Commanders to Determine Psychological Fitness**

| Peers and Family Members | Service Members, Themselves |
|---|---|
| ☐ Service member has <u>not</u> demonstrated any unsafe behaviors, such as strong suicidal thoughts or violent impulses.<br><br>☐ Service member is not drinking excessively or engaging in any other dangerous behavior.<br><br>☐ Service member appears to those most familiar with him or her to have returned to his or her normal or usual self.<br><br>☐ Peers and family members are comfortable living and working with Service member. | ☐ Service member feels confident in his or her ability to perform effectively and remain well.<br><br>☐ Service member is motivated to remain on active duty and deploy. |

# APPENDIX L

# SUICIDE PREVENTION

Suicide is the ultimate failure of stress control. When a Service member dies by suicide, the needless loss of life is a tragedy. Family members and friends who are left behind must grapple with the painful questions of why and how. The loss of a Marine or Sailor is deeply felt by all those who remain behind. Why did this happen? How can a future tragedy be averted? What lessons can be learned and used to prevent another loss? What actions were taken or not taken and what could have been done to identify Marines and Sailors who most needed help and support?

> Suicide is the ultimate failure of stress control.

The most likely Marine to die by suicide corresponds to Marine Corps institutional demographics—male, 18 to 25 years old, between the ranks of E-1 and E-5 (private to sergeant). In the Navy, suicides are most common between the ranks of E-3 and E-6 (third class to first class petty officers). Suicide rates in both Services appear to be related to overall operating tempo or operational stress load and do not appear to fluctuate by deployment history. The most common stressors associated with suicide are romantic or family relationship problems, work-related problems, pending adverse legal or administrative actions, physical health problems, and job dissatisfaction. Despite the demographics, no one is immune and an at-risk member cannot be predicted.

There are almost always multiple stressors and risk factors in each suicide case. Suicide prevention involves initiatives that approach the problem from multiple angles. The five core COSC and OSC leadership functions play a significant role in addressing solutions to suicide awareness and prevention. Strengthening, mitigation, identification, treatment, and reintegration are crucial to suicide prevention in any command. Leaders must build resilience in all aspects of their Marines' and Sailors' lives, reduce unnecessary stressors, identify problems as early as possible, ensure appropriate early intervention or treatment to resolve problems before they become overwhelming, and ensure that Service members remain full and functional members of their units.

# Strengthen

An ounce of prevention is worth a pound of cure. Strong, resilient Marines and Sailors have multiple options for dealing with problems and are less likely to become overwhelmed to the point of suicide. They are capable of responding effectively and confidently to problems and threats. They have strong families, units, and leaders that engender trust and a sense of safety in seeking help. They have the confidence, willpower, fortitude, and vision to see beyond the stress of the moment. At the crucial moment, they can answer, "Yes, I can handle this problem." They help each other, watching for someone having problems, offering to help before their problems become larger and seemingly beyond solution. They have confidence and trust that "Yes, *we* can handle this problem."

# Mitigate

A crucial role of leaders in suicide prevention is to reduce as much *unnecessary* stress as possible. Unnecessary hassles and frustrations drain crucial coping resources needed for dealing with the everyday conflicts of life, such as relationships, job issues, and accountability for actions. Though military service must be demanding so that Service members keep their edge, some stressors do not sharpen motivation and skills, but serve to make them dull and depleted. Leaders must be careful to constantly assess the impact of their demands on Service members and their families. Firm and fair leadership is respected and inspiring, but capricious and irresponsible leadership is toxic. Whenever possible, leaders should ensure that Service members have the training, skills, resources, and time to deal with their personal problems. The balance between allowing Service members time to take care of themselves versus the needs of the mission at hand is a risk management decision leaders must constantly make, weighing long-term versus immediate readiness.

# Identify

One of the most critical functions of leadership is to identify Marines, Sailors, and families who have having problems that may be affecting their personal readiness as early as possible and before they become overwhelming. Sometimes this can be difficult. Leaders often want to give Service members the benefit of the doubt with the hope that the problems will resolve on their own. They may not want to intrude; however, early identification does not necessarily mean immediate intrusive intervention. Rather, it can mean having awareness and maintaining a watchful waiting, assessing when the problem and the person involved are ready for intervention.

Leaders must create a command climate in which early identification is perceived by those involved as having the best interests of Service members in mind. It must be perceived as nonpunitive, with the goal of helping them get back to the full readiness and function they desire. The help must be perceived as safe to accept so Service members don't have incentive to cover up or deny. They must understand that the right thing to do is to ask for help and answer honestly on deployment health assessments. Unit leaders and Service members must be up to date on suicide prevention training and know what to watch for, ask, and do in sensitive situations. The ultimate bad outcome is when the Service member feels there is nowhere to turn, rejects offers of help from leaders and peers, and continues to spiral into hopelessness. The early warning signs of problems are those of the Yellow Zone in the stress continuum model, when a leader can still make a big difference directly. Once the Orange Zone indicator light comes on, however, it is time for the Service member to be referred to professional medical intervention.

> Leaders must create a command climate in which early identification is perceived by those involved as having the best interests of Service members in mind.

## Treat

In suicide prevention (as in COSC and OSC), generally, early and effective treatment of Yellow Zone stress reactions and Orange Zone stress injuries is impossible without the direct leadership of unit commanders and the active participation of their chains of command, families, and individual Service members. With effective early intervention by leaders, many problems can be solved before they require professional intervention. Successful early intervention will increase confidence in unit leadership and reduce the stigma of asking for help. Waiting until problems escalate reduces the probability of successful resolution and increases the risk of suicidal behavior. It is crucial to know when a Service member's problems have progressed beyond the scope of leadership intervention and need to be referred for professional help. Of course, when a Service member reports suicide-related thoughts, an immediate professional assessment is warranted.

Leaders must also be aware that suicide risk often increases as help is received and mood improves. Sustained attention during treatment is necessary for reducing risk even when things appear to be improving.

## Reintegrate

The process of reintegrating the Service member into the routine of the unit is a significant part of COSC, OSC, and stress first aid. The Service member must regain hope and honor. The stress first aid actions of connect, competence, and confidence allow leaders to reconnect affected Service members with their trusted peers and encourage peer support by giving them meaningful work and opportunities for success until a sense of competence is restored. Reintegration is needed after the Service member has received professional help or any time he may have lost his confidence or that of his peers.

When intervention has been early enough to prevent suicidal behavior, reintegration is part of restrengthening—letting Service members know that their leaders value them and have confidence and trust that they will recover. Reintegration in a prejudice-free environment is crucial to restoration of full readiness.

## Resources

The following more specific information on suicide prevention is available online:

Marine Corps Suicide Prevention Web site: http://www.usmc-mccs.org/suicideprevent

Marine Corps Leaders Guide for Managing Marines in Distress: http://www.usmc-mccs.org/leadersguide

Navy Suicide Prevention Web site: http://www.npc.navy.mil/CommandSupport/SuicidePrevention/

Navy Environmental Health Center Suicide Prevention Web site: http://www-nehc.med.navy.mil/hp/suicide

Navy Leader's Guide for Managing Personnel in Distress: http://www-nmcphc.med.navy.mil/lguide

# APPENDIX M

# INDIVIDUAL AUGMENTATION PROGRAM CHALLENGES

Individual augmentees face challenges that are unlike those of Service members who deploy with their own units. These challenges place them at increased risk for Yellow Zone stress reactions and Orange Zone stress injuries. Challenges may include assimilation into the receiving unit, premature and sudden termination of bonds formed with the unit upon redeployment, reintegration with the parent unit, and lack of presence and support from those with shared experiences after returning home. Adding to these challenges are the additional sources of stress faced by individual augmentees who are assigned to deploy in a role for which they have had little or no previous training, possibly with a unit from a different military service with unfamiliar customs and practices. With proper awareness and sensitivity to issues particular to individual augmentees, leaders can mitigate risk and optimize unit function.

## Adapting the Five COSC and OSC Leadership Functions for Individual Augmentees

The five core COSC and OSC leadership functions can relate to individual augmentees in the following ways:

- *Strengthen.* Optimal functioning in any military environment, especially in combat, requires Marines and Sailors to have good working relationships based on mutual trust and respect. The process of building unit cohesion is thought to shield warriors from COS and begins when a Service member joins a unit and is given realistic training by solid and competent leadership. One of the biggest obstacles for the individual augmentee is joining a unit late in the deployment cycle and integrating with other warriors who may be resentful. Leaders should pay close attention to the mission planning and assimilation processes, ensuring that individual augmentees join the unit at the earliest possible time and integrate with their unit. Identifying "battle buddies" during training can protect Service members against stress injuries as can practicing Navy or Marine Corps customs and traditions when deployed with a unit from another Service. Examples include establishing a quarterdeck or decorating living quarters in a Navy or Marine Corp theme.

- *Mitigate*. Social support at home, whether it is the family, the parent command, or a Reserve center, plays a large role in COSC and OSC. In some cases, leaders support Sailors and Marines while they deal with crises that arise at home during the deployment, such as illness of a loved one, relationship problems, or lack of communication. On the other hand, leaders should take every opportunity to promote Service members' abilities to communicate with people back home who provide meaningful support. A time of potentially great stress for individual augmentees is at redeployment, when the abrupt termination of strong bonds with members of the deployed unit can result in grief and loss and can aggravate stress reactions or injuries. Leaders should respect these bonds and facilitate a smooth, appreciative separation with command sanctioned hail and farewell ceremonies. As much as possible, leaders should preserve cohesion with individual augmentees by encouraging their Marines and Sailors to maintain contact with them after they return to their parent commands. Parent commanders of returning individual augmentees have to be especially aware of individual augmentee challenges and provide an understanding environment, affording opportunities to the individual augmentee to vent, discuss, and share knowledge with others.

- *Identify*. Individual augmentees may depend on their unit chains of command and peers to monitor their stressors and stress zones even more than other Service members because individual augmentees are less well-known and are less likely to divulge personal information to others whom they don't yet trust. The primary responsibility for monitoring stress and identifying stress zones for individual augmentees lies with the commanding officer of the parent unit; however, tracking and following up with individual augmentees can be challenging because some individual augmentees will receive a permanent change of station move after returning. Automated tracking methods independent of duty station should be perfected to help both losing and gaining parent commands with this process. As much as possible, leaders should personally conduct turnover of individual augmentees with the receiving command to ensure a seamless transition.

- *Treat.* Once a severe Yellow Zone stress reaction or Orange Zone stress injury is identified in an individual augmentee, its treatment is much the same as it would be for an organic unit member. The same seven Cs of stress first aid apply as do the same medical and pastoral care principals. Care and treatment of individual augmentees are uniquely challenged by the obstacles to social support and to the continuity of all treatment approaches after redeployment or returning to the parent unit. Leaders of the parent command may know nothing about the during-deployment stressors or stress zones.
- *Reintegrate.* Reintegration is also challenging for individual augmentees who experience Yellow, Orange, or Red Zone stress during and after deployments. As they recover, they have to be mentored back to full competence and confidence within their deployed unit; moreover, after they redeploy, individual augmentees must regain their competence and confidence with their parent unit and their families. Leaders in the deployed unit should help their Marines or Sailors prepare to reintegrate with their postdeployment lives and work. Leaders in the parent and deployed units communicate stress zone information about the Service member to provide an uninterrupted reintegration. Leaders should also give Marines and Sailors a chance to reflect upon their experiences and honor and recognize their service during and after the transition. For many individual augmentees, such recognition and time to reflect is absent upon return, which can cause bitterness and moral conflict.

# Challenges for Family Members of Individual Augmentees

Families of individual augmentees sometimes fall through a large crack between the family readiness programs and services of their parent and deployed units. It may be difficult for the spouses of individual augmentees to build cohesion with other unit spouses or with family readiness organizations when they live thousands of miles away from both. Leaders of both parent and deployed commands should recognize the unique stressors that individual augmentee families experience and work with the unit's family readiness officers (FROs) to provide outreach and support. Monthly command family letters to include individual augmentee families, availability of state-of-the-art internet and phone connections, and fast mail service may be provided by the deployed command to maintain family mental health.

# MARINE CORPS OPERATIONAL
# STRESS CONTROL AND READINESS PROGRAM

In 1999, 2d Marine Division developed and fielded a new type of partnership between warfighters, mental health professionals, and chaplains—Operational Stress Control and Readiness (OSCAR) program—that differed from any previous military mental health effort. It assigns mental health personnel as organic assets in ground combat units at the division level, rather than attaching them to external medical treatment facilities or combat stress teams.

Psychiatrists, psychologists, and psychiatric technicians who are part of the OSCAR program are organic to the military units they support in the same way battalion surgeons, corpsmen, and chaplains are organic to their Marine operational units. Ideally, OSCAR MHPs train with their Marines prior to deployment, accompany their Marines into forward operational areas during deployment, and continue to provide support to their Marines after they return from deployment. The OSCAR program bridges the cultural gap between warfighters and mental health professionals by drawing professionals as fully as possible into the culture and life of the military units they support and making them more members of the "family" than outsiders. The intent of this effort is to reduce the stigma of mental health care through familiarity and shared adversity.

The OSCAR program's mental health personnel have been continually assigned to ground combat element units since the OSCAR pilot project began in 2004. In 2007, the commanding generals of all three MEFs jointly requested that OSCAR be institutionalized, staffed, and supported by Headquarters, Marine Corps (HQMC) and Navy Medicine. In 2008, a permanent OSCAR mental health program became one of the priorities of the Marine Corps Combat Development Command and the Chief of Naval Personnel. It authorized 26 mental health professionals and 29 paraprofessional psychiatric technician corpsmen (NEC 8485) to the Marine infantry divisions and regiments of the active and Reserve forces to be filled by the end of the 2011 fiscal year. In the interim, Navy Medicine continues to fill OSCAR mental health requirements for deploying units on an ad hoc basis.

Marine leaders quickly recognized that, although this was a good start, there would still be insufficient MHPs to prevent, identify, and manage the growing number of Marines and Sailors with COS problems across the Corps. In 2009, the Assistant Commandant of the Marine Corps directed the extension of OSCAR capabilities down to the infantry battalion and company levels, without requiring additional mental health resources, by providing special OSCAR team training to existing medical and religious ministry personnel (OSCAR extenders) as well as selected warfighters (OSCAR mentors). The goal of the training was to build Marine-led OSCAR teams of mentors, extenders, and mental health personnel for each infantry battalion, each with the basic knowledge, skills, attitudes, and tools required to help the unit commander prevent, identify, and manage COS problems as early as possible.

The OSCAR capability is now being applied across all the operating forces (ground combat divisions, air wings, and logistic groups) and is also being developed for the supporting establishment and family communities. As a result, the focus of OSCAR has changed dramatically, from originally embedding mental health assets in infantry divisions to what is now a comprehensive line-led tool for leaders that is supported by medical, religious ministry, and mental health assets from a variety of sources.

## OSCAR Concept of Operations

OSCAR teams are formed at the battalion level (units of approximately 1000 Marines) across the Corps. Each unit trains a team of approximately 50 OSCAR mentors, derived from both the battalion headquarters unit and subordinate units; moreover, it uses supporting extenders and MHPs from internal or local sources, as available. The team's task is to help the unit commander prevent, identify, and manage COS problems as early as possible.

The OSCAR program brings mentors, extenders, and MHPs together for six hours of training. The training includes COSC awareness, application of the stress continuum, the five core leader functions, AARs as COSC tools, listening skills, early intervention strategies, operational risk management issues related to stress, coordination between leaders and medical providers, tools for building resilience, mitigation strategies, determination of psychological readiness for deployment, and a leader's panel discussion of personal experiences with COS. The panel is added to the training as an opportunity for leaders to demonstrate to their subordinates that it is acceptable to talk about COS. The COSC/OSCAR professional specialty training for medical and religious ministry personnel (extenders and MHPs) is provided by Marine Corps field medical training schools, as well as other venues provided by BUMED and the Chief of Chaplains.

The OSCAR mentors consist of selected Marines with combat zone deployment experience, who are strong role models and are willing to assist and mentor other Marines with COS problems. The battalion headquarters element would typically assign its executive officer, sergeant major, and selected Marines to serve as OSCAR mentors; likewise, each company in the battalion would typically assign its executive officer, first sergeant, and selected Marines. Mentors are responsible for identifying, supporting, and advising Marines with COS issues as early as possible, providing leadership through example and referring them to OSCAR extenders and MHPs when problems persist. The reason for putting Marines on the front line is not only to empower leaders to help Marines recognize and recover from stress problems and get back in the fight more quickly, but also to free up MHPs from taking care of cases not requiring mental health treatment. Putting Marines on the front line also reduces stigma by giving Marines initial contacts they can trust—their brothers in arms who have "been there and done that."

The OSCAR extenders consist of medical staff, chaplains, licensed counselors, corpsmen, religious support specialists, and other professionals who "extend" the capabilities of OSCAR MHPs by bridging the gap between MHPs and Marine mentors. The individuals assigned or invited to be part of the battalion team will depend on the type of unit and local support available. For example, OSCAR teams in infantry battalions have battalion medical and religious ministry assets plus company corpsmen organic to them; these would typically be assigned to participate with their respective battalion OSCAR teams. Most supporting establishment commands, however, do not have such assets organic to their command and must rely on external resources, such as installation medical and religious ministry services, for support. Some remote commands must rely on other military services or civilian resources to assist their teams. In most cases these battalions would be advised to invite providers with whom they have or would like to have a good working relationship to be part of their OSCAR team to facilitate familiarization and mutual understanding of missions.

Extenders provide professional support within their respective scopes of practice. Examples include medical treatment of sleep problems, anxiety, depression, counseling for marital problems, anger management, burnout, loss, inner conflict, anxiety, depression, and other noncomplicated mental health issues commonly addressed by primary care physicians, chaplains, and licensed counselors. Corpsmen and religious support specialists have limited specialty skills as extenders but function as peer mentors alongside their Marines, being similar in age and rank and closely trusted.

The OSCAR mental health personnel consists of psychiatrists, psychologists, mental health nurse practitioners, and licensed clinical social workers embedded in operational units to provide formal mental health services. The individuals assigned or invited to be part of the battalion team also depend on the type of unit and support available. Each infantry division generally includes three mental health professionals and four psychological technicians on their table of organization. Each infantry regiment typically includes two mental health professionals and two psychological technicians, all available on a shared basis to their respective battalions. However, outside of the infantry divisions, commands must generally rely on external mental health resources, such as installation mental health services, for support. Some remote commands must rely on other military services or civilian resources to assist their teams. In such cases, these commands would be advised to invite external MHPs with whom they have or would like to have a good working relationship to be an informal part of their OSCAR team and facilitate familiarization and mutual understanding of missions.

Mental health personnel assigned to operational units provide not only direct clinical services, but also spend a significant portion of their time in the field with the Marines they support during training and deployment. Organic OSCAR mental health personnel augment the following capabilities for their commanders:

- Psychological health surveillance of unit members and units as a whole.
- Preventive psychological health training.

- Early interventions to promote recovery for individuals and units from life-threat or losses.
- Clinical mental health services in forward operational environments where such services would be otherwise unavailable.
- Professional coordination of comprehensive mental health care services in garrison before and after deployments to ensure readiness.
- Clinical mental health services in garrison as an adjunct to those provided by medical treatment facilities.
- Psychological health support for medical and religious ministry personnel who are at high risk for stress-related problems.

The OSCAR mental health personnel also support their command's psychological health through the following specific functions and tasks:

- Advise commanders and other members of the chain of command on their leadership of psychological health, resilience, and COSC.
- Become known to their Marines and trusted by them through repeated contact and the sharing of adversity.
- Learn as much as possible about the stressors their Marines face, how they normally cope with stressors, and how Marine leaders manage and mitigate stressors.
- Educate and train Marines and Marine leaders in evidence-based methods for preventing, identifying, and managing adverse stress reactions.
- Consult with primary care medical officers and corpsmen on the management of adverse stress reactions that require further care.
- Consult with Marine Corps chaplains regarding their stress management functions.
- Consult with military leaders on the management of unit-level stress challenges.
- Work closely with their command element, maintaining an awareness of ongoing operations and paying particular attention to events and operations likely to generate COS casualties.

To be effective, the OSCAR MHPs cannot retreat to a familiar clinical setting surrounded by medical and mental health colleagues. The OSCAR MHP must learn to be comfortable in the world of the Marine. Similarly, Marine leaders must learn to communicate with their mental health professionals, consider their guidance, and incorporate the information and technologies they bring into the culture of the unit. Because of the shortage of mental health manpower resources, OSCAR team members must also balance the competing priorities of providing preventive services in operational or training environments with providing direct clinical care.

# APPENDIX O

# SPECIAL PSYCHIATRIC RAPID INTERVENTION TEAMS

Life at sea is inherently dangerous. Despite continuous development of technology that improves the capability of modern Sailors to operate in the air, on the sea, and below the surface, disasters at sea can generate stress reactions like those of Marines in combat. This observation was reinforced during the 1970s when the US Navy experienced several major disasters.

As thousands of Vietnam veterans manifested the newly recognized condition of PTSD, two major naval mishaps prompted the Navy mental health community to develop a concept for early intervention. In 1975, the USS Belknap and the USS John F. Kennedy collided, resulting in significant loss of life and extensive damage to both ships. In 1977, another collision occurred in Spain. As a result, the Psychiatry Department at Portsmouth Naval Hospital—now called the Naval Medical Center, Portsmouth—saw many patients with related stress symptoms and developed a plan for early intervention. They used the same concepts developed to treat stress in combat for early intervention with disasters at sea and created the special psychiatric rapid intervention teams (SPRINTs).

## Organization and Mission

In 1983, SPRINTs were formally chartered under BUMED Instruction 6440.6, *Mobile Medical Augmentation Readiness Team (MMART) Manual*. Navy SPRINTs are formally organized at Bethesda, MD; Portsmouth, VA; and San Diego, CA, with some informally organized teams at various overseas locations. A SPRINT mission is formally initiated in accordance with BUMED Instruction 3301.3A, *Medical Operations Center (MOC)*. Since their inception, SPRINTs have not only provided intervention in maritime mishaps, but also stability and contingency operations, terrorist attacks, and natural disasters. The teams consist of two psychiatrists, two clinical psychologists, one chaplain, one psychiatric nurse, and four hospital corpsmen psychiatric technicians. The mission of the SPRINT is for its members to—

- Be trained and immediately available in the event of a contingency.
- Provide assessment of the psychological effects of traumatic stress.
- Provide direct support to individuals and units affected by the traumatic event.
- Provide brief psychiatric treatment as needed.
- Provide consultation to commanders and leaders on how to mitigate the negative impact of the event.

# Intervention Strategies

Team members are expected to be competent in their respective disciplines and well-versed on the latest information in crisis intervention techniques and treatment strategies for acute stress and PTSD. Interventions should be consistent with general Navy and Marine Corps doctrine on COSC and OSC and with the stress continuum model. During the 1980s and 1990s, the technique of critical incident stress debriefing was developed to help emergency services workers, such as firefighters, paramedics, and police officers address particularly stressful events. The military attempted to adopt it for use in its interventions, but now discourages it because it has not been proven effective in controlled trials and evidence indicates that it may be harmful. Instead, the current focus is on providing command consultation, psycho-educational intervention, and psychological first aid. The team assists the command in developing a strategy to mitigate the impact of the event on the entire organization; provides timely, targeted, and useful information for command members; and treats only those individuals who are in acute distress. Even for individual treatment, every attempt is made to avoid labeling or diagnosing too early. Rather, the individual is encouraged to mobilize his own resources to enhance recovery and restore functioning.

In addition to being knowledgeable about acute intervention theory and techniques, team members must be able to operate in diverse settings where they could be deployed. These settings include surface ships, submarines, and aviation locations as well as with SEABEES [Navy construction engineers] and Marines. Team members must also be knowledgeable and comfortable with various Navy systems, organizations, and structural issues that will affect how well a command withstands the impact of a stressful event.

During war time, most SPRINTs are dormant due to pressing demands for mental health manpower to deploy with other operational platforms; however, the valuable concepts, skills, and techniques developed through the Navy SPRINT's experiences in peacetime educate the wider Navy mental health community, improving the stress intervention and treatment of the operating forces.

Navy SPRINTs continue to be a useful tool to assist commands affected by severely stressful events. The Navy SPRINT concept will continue to evolve with the Navy mental health community to meet the challenges and threats of an ever-changing world.

# APPENDIX P

# HUMANITARIAN ASSISTANCE AND DISASTER RELIEF/RESPONSE CHALLENGES

Global concerns have changed remarkably since 2001. Responding to new and emerging threats, theater security cooperation programs dictate that naval forces operate across a wide range of environments and circumstances. Included among these initiatives are missions designed to shape peacekeeping and influence nation building. The Marine Corps calls these programs *disaster relief*, while the Navy uses the term *disaster response*.

Each time a hospital ship is deployed or a warship responds to a natural disaster, the Navy takes on the "public relations" role to change hearts and minds, influence public opinion, and project a positive image of the United States. When a nation's own disaster relief/response capability is overwhelmed, as in 2005 when a 9.0 earthquake-triggered tsunami slammed into Banda Aceh, Indonesia, Sailors and Marines rushed to the aid of the stricken country with medical assistance, civil affairs, civil engineering, logistics and supplies, and water purification assets.

Regardless of the size or complexity of the assistance mission, many Sailors and Marines are exposed to levels of human suffering and devastation that may lead to stress reactions or injuries. Leaders will be able to assess their Sailors and Marines more appropriately if they have a basic understanding of the two levels of disaster relief/response.

## Disaster Relief/Response Phases and Challenges

Planners divide disaster relief/response initiatives into two phases—acute emergency and reconsolidation/postemergency. During the acute emergency phase, relief workers and emergency responders provide basic needs, such as food, drinkable water, sanitation, shelter, basic health care services, and security. They also provide stress first aid and enhanced social support systems to manage stress injuries noted among the local population.

During the reconsolidation phase, relief workers restore and provide general health care services. They also reconstruct roads, bridges, and communications systems. Responding mental health teams work with primary care providers and other health care staff, while community workers conduct outreach activities. Complex disasters—such as those with existing conflict, population displacement, or food scarcity—create a greater risk for military responders. Different regions of a country may fluctuate between acute and postemergency phases during a complex disaster.

Seriously traumatized populations may significantly affect military responders, including aviation personnel, cargo handlers, Navy construction engineers, civil engineers, corpsmen, physicians, nurses, dentists, and nonmedical support personnel. During both phases of the disaster scenario, self-care may need to wait though survivor guilt may slowly numb the ability of the responders to monitor themselves or, more importantly, to self-refer. Responders may experience vicarious trauma or compassion fatigue due to the seemingly never-ending needs of the victims or from repeatedly listening to stories that echo the magnitude of the devastation.

Leaders must watch for secondary traumatic stress and burnout as well as wear-and-tear stress injuries, which are more likely to occur after a period of time and are more common during the reconsolidation phase. All reactions must be anticipated, identified, and appropriately managed.

# Leader Actions

For all Service members, stress first aid remains the mainstay of self-care and buddy care. One of the most important services an individual can do for someone who has been directly or indirectly traumatized is to be a supportive, nonjudgmental, active listener. Predeployment COSC and OSC training is warranted for all deploying Marines and Sailors. As they respond to a natural or manmade disaster, leaders must prepare their troops to expect pervasive misfortune, suffering, loss, and their own possible reacting (Yellow Zone) behaviors. Injured (Orange Zone) behaviors may result from repeated and prolonged exposure to such despair and are likely to be seen in individuals with prior trauma history.

Service members ashore responding to disaster scenarios and exposed to unrelenting stress should be rotated back onboard ship or out of the impact area for rest, recreation, or even just a hot shower if not available elsewhere. Exercise is vital to healthy coping as is a balanced work-rest cycle. Given the intensity of operations, AARs led by tactical leaders provide the necessary framework for understanding, processing, and education.

# THE ROLE OF RELIGIOUS MINISTRY PERSONNEL

The religious ministry team (RMT), composed of at least one chaplain and one religious program specialist or chaplain's assistant, may be an integrated, organic part of the Navy or Marine Corps unit or assigned by higher headquarters to deliver religious ministry to a command. Chaplains are uniquely qualified to deliver specific care, such as counseling. They help Service members with personal and relationship issues that may be outside a religious context. Such counseling is most effective when religious ministry personnel share life and experiences with the unit. Chaplains build strong relationships that are distinguished by their immediate presence, confidentiality, professional wisdom, and genuine respect for human beings. While their work in care and referral increases with the severity of their Service member's stress injuries, chaplains work with medical personnel to help leaders build resilience in units through community support programs, training, ministering to Service members in their workspaces, and advising commanders. The RMTs are also the frontline professional response-care—assessment and referral— experts when Service members are reacting to stressful environments. The RMT's primary mission is to provide ministry and pastoral care to the troops and offer faith, assurance, and hope. The RMT provides field services and pastoral counsel and facilitates religious practices, building resilience before the mission and helping Service members integrate their experiences with their lives after deployment.

## Spiritual Guidance

Personal resources that aid resilience are often based on faith, religious beliefs, and spiritual values. In combat, Service members may either show increased interest in their religious beliefs or lose faith during its chaos. In the latter case, Service members can experience the inner conflict, fear, despair, and hopelessness that may eventually lead to a stress injury or illness. Chaplains are a source of direction and stability for Service members who experience these dilemmas and seek to refocus their personal beliefs and spiritual values.

## Pastoral Counseling and Referrals

Unique to the command, chaplains are required to maintain confidentiality when a Service member seeks out his counsel and care. Chaplains are not in the unit chain of command and afford a nonthreatening place for returning Marines or Sailors to discuss important life and spiritual issues.

Chaplains work with unit and attached physicians, psychiatrists, and psychologists. While not expected to deliver counseling with the same expertise as mental health providers, a chaplain's pastoral care and counseling may make invaluable contributions to the command in caring for those in need. Chaplains are also the first line referral source to higher levels of care when issues are beyond their training, so they have the unique role of being a buffer for those unsure if they need higher levels of care.

The RMTs maintain constant interaction with family crisis support services at home. If operational events during deployment create crises of anxiety or grief in family members, family crisis support services can be immediately requested through the facility chaplain and MCCS or the Navy Fleet and Family Support Center. Coordination between the involved RMT and the local MCCS or Navy Fleet and Family Support Center office is crucial to successfully resolve deployment-related problems.

## Ministry of Presence

The RMT's presence in training events and unit life make it a trusted resource when Service members need help. The RMT should be present with Service members during training and, especially, deployment. The chaplain and religious program specialist can be a calming influence on Service members and can help them strengthen or regain values important to them. Chaplains can help mitigate combat stress and misconduct by—

- Being present with the Service members and deploying with the unit.
- Visiting Service members in work and living areas.

- Providing opportunities for private and group prayer and worship.
- Supplying personal religious articles and materials.
- Reading the scriptures with Service members.
- Providing sacraments.

# Counseling for Grief and Inner Conflict

Understanding COS and the unique role that spirituality and religion play in promoting holistic health are essential when dealing with grief and inner conflict. Grief and inner conflict injuries are areas where chaplains are uniquely qualified to offer assistance to Marines and Sailors in distress.

War zone trauma produces both positive and negative feelings about God, religion, and spirituality that trained chaplains are best positioned to address before, during, and after combat or operational experiences. These experiences change all Marines and Sailors biologically, psychologically, socially, and spiritually. Medical personnel can address the former two, but only chaplains are trained to address the latter two. Chaplains are particularly focused on personal, relational, and familial health and well-being, both by training and by nature, and are adept at partnering with other helping professionals. Spirituality and religion frequently provide "safe havens" in which to explore concerns over combat and operational experiences, especially for those who are suffering from any degree of combat stress and are reluctant to admit it.

# Delivery of Stress First Aid

Chaplains also train Service members in stress first aid and the buddy system and can provide a higher level of skill in performing it when needed. If possible, chaplains should use the same programs taught at professional development training courses and offered through the Marine Operational Stress Training (MOST) program. Using these programs avoids quality variance based on individual agendas and ensures that all Marines and Sailors are afforded the best possible evidence-based information to aid reintegration with society and families at home.

# Role of RMTs in the Five
# Core Functions of COSC and OSC

The established relationship between RMTs and the commands they support promotes trust with the troops. As integral members of their commands, RMTs are trained and ready to respond to the needs of Service members experiencing combat or other operational stress. A person-oriented resource, the team ministers across the continuum of stress zones, but mostly in the Yellow and Orange Zones where Marines and Sailors have the potential to be returned to full duty quickly after rest. Chaplains provide unique support in each of the five COSC and OSC leadership functions:

- *Strengthen.* Chaplains provide and facilitate religious services, rituals, and pastoral care to strengthen individuals in their everyday life. Participation in religion has been shown to increase resiliency of individuals who have been involved in stressful events. Chaplains convey the strength and hope that religious convictions and faith may provide to Service members, especially in a combat or operational setting, regardless of faith group or denomination. This enthusiastic, inclusive ministry greatly enhances the morale of the unit.
- *Mitigate.* When a unit is involved in a combat engagement, AARs may help Service members to make sense of the event and calm excess stress. While the RMT helps Service members to rebuild their emotional, psychological, and spiritual strength, the team members are also helped by being available to counsel affected Marines and Sailors. Their ongoing direct religious ministry includes providing/coordinating the availability of worship services, sacraments, rites, and services/ceremonies honoring the dead—all designed to help individuals return to normal functioning.
- *Identify.* The RMTs help commanders identify Service members experiencing COS. Chaplains work closely with the medical officer and are trained to recognize the signs, symptoms, and zones of combat stress and to provide religious support to Service members in need of pastoral care. As a result, they are also able to identify and to refer individuals who require a higher level of care. The RMTs also continuously assess spiritual needs to provide or to facilitate the appropriate religious ministry.

- *Treat*. Chaplains recognize stress problems across the stress continuum model, but mainly work with Yellow Zone Marines and Sailors. Very few chaplains have the training and expertise to provide treatment of Marines past the Yellow Zone. Their role in the injured and ill zones is to make referrals and then to visit Marines and Sailors who have been referred for treatment or are resting or recuperating.
- *Reintegrate*. The RMT is still with the unit when a Marine or Sailor returns to it and can assist with his reintegration. Chaplains can be a great source of strength and encouragement for returning Marines and Sailors.

# APPENDIX R

# THE ROLE OF UNIT MEDICAL PERSONNEL IN MARINE CORPS COMBAT AND OPERATIONAL STRESS CONTROL

The incidence of COS can increase when operating tempo is high due to multiple "back to back" deployments/extended combat operations. As unit medical personnel, such as battalion/ regimental surgeons, independent duty corpsmen (IDC), and field medical technicians (8404 corpsmen), provide the primary care for the Marines of their unit, they most likely will be the first to evaluate and treat members for COS problems. They are also uniquely positioned to help prevent COS by providing COSC classes to help build resiliency within unit members.

The mission of medical personnel regarding Marine Corps COSC requires that it be prepared to assist in the prevention of COS within the unit and identify and provide initial evaluation and treatment for COS. The mission also requires that medical personnel obtain a mental health professional consultation from or formally refer Service members to a mental health professional when the severity of the COS is beyond the scope of the operational medicine privileges in order to preserve the combat power of the unit.

## Supporting Units and Personnel

Other personnel available to unit medical personnel include the unit chaplain, who can provide COSC classes and other assistance to those experiencing COS; the division psychiatrist; combat stress department of the combat logistics battalion; the OSCAR team; the mental health department of the local military treatment facility (MTF); and the unit FRO. Mental health providers assigned to Fleet Marine Force units and MHPs and educators assigned to the MCCS and Semper Fit are available to assist in providing unit COSC classes. The unit FRO is also available to provide assistance with and training for the families of their Marines and Sailors.

# Concept of Operations

Marine Corps philosophy, Marine Corps Bulletin (MCBul) 6490, *Combat Operational Stress Control (COSC) Program*, emphasizes prevention over treatment and wellness over injury, so unit medical personnel assist the commander by providing the unit with MOST in connection with the unit deployment cycle. They identify those with COS, evaluate and treat them using unit-level personnel and assets, and, as necessary, seek the assistance of an MHP for guidance or formally refer the patient. Unit medical personnel, particularly the corpsmen, have served "shoulder to shoulder" with Marines during peacetime and war and as unit safety representatives; they have their "finger on the pulse" of their units. They train with Marines during field exercises prior to deployment, deploy together, reside in the same barracks or berthing space, and evaluate/treat all of their other medical conditions in garrison and in the field. Accordingly, unit medical personnel are leaders in the management of COS.

# Unit Medical Officer Tasks

Regimental, group, and battalion flight surgeons and IDC must—

- Attend a HQMC-approved COSC for health care providers training program to become proficient with the Marine Corps COSC program as outlined in MCBul 6490, the stress continuum model, and the stress continuum decision flowchart. Unit medical providers must be able to use the approved COS-prevention techniques, provide initial intervention and treatment according to their particular scope of practice, and know when it is appropriate to seek the assistance of or refer the patient to a mental health professional both in garrison and while deployed.
- Advise their commanding officer on the Marine Corps COSC program.
- Inform their commanding officer about all Marines in the unit who are having significant difficulty managing COS using the stress continuum model.

- Update the commanding officer on the status of all mental health patients from the unit who are being treated and provide recommendations on their fitness for duty/deployment.
- Ensure senior medical officers train the unit's junior medical officers, physician assistants, IDC, and corpsmen on their roles and responsibilities in the Marine Corps COSC program and its implementation while adhering to the aforementioned references, which can also be found on the HQMC, Manpower and Reserve Affairs (M&RA) COSC Web site (www.manpower.usmc.mil/cosc).
- Provide or coordinate the training of the unit's Marines, leaders, and families on the "deployment phase-specific" COSC topics with the unit chaplain, unit OSCAR team, or division psychiatrist as required by the aforementioned references.
- Understand the local and organic mental health resources, such as the division psychiatrist, OSCAR team, deployment health clinic, MTF mental health department, MCCS, Semper Fit, Military OneSource, and the M&RA COSC Web site, that are available to the unit while in garrison and while on deployment in order to properly educate the unit, advise the leadership, and ensure timely mental health referrals for their personnel.

## Unit Field Medical Technicians (8404 Corpsmen) Tasks

Responsibilities of medical technicians include—

- Becoming proficient with the COSC program, the stress continuum model, and the stress continuum decision flowchart by attending a HQMC-approved COSC for health care providers training program or training received from the unit medical officer or IDC. Corpsmen must be able to use the approved COS-prevention techniques, be capable of providing initial intervention in accordance with their unit medical officer's guidance, and know when to seek the assistance of their medical officer or a mental health professional when the unit medical officer is not available.
- Keeping the unit medical officer and unit leader informed of all Marines or Sailors having significant difficulty managing COS. The unit may be a company, platoon, section, Marine military transition team, squad, or crew.
- Advising the unit leader on the COSC program.

- Ensuring that junior corpsmen are trained on the COSC program and that they know their roles and responsibilities in its implementation at their unit.
- Providing training for Marines and Sailors from their unit on the "deployment phase-specific" COSC topics required by MCBul 6490 and found on the HQMC M&RA COSC Web site.
- Knowing the local and organic mental health resources that are available to the unit while in garrison or while deployed to properly educate their unit, advise their leadership, and help ensure timely mental health referrals. Some resources include the division psychiatrist, OSCAR team, deployment health clinic, MTF mental health department, MCCS, Semper Fit, Military OneSource, and the M&RA COSC Web site.

## Coordinating Instructions

Educational and training materials used to teach the COSC program adhere to the MCBul 6490 and may be found on the M&RA COSC Web site. To be flexible in varied operating environments and still meet the MCBul 6490 requirements, unit medical departments—at the discretion of their respective commanding officers—may also produce briefs or training materials, which integrate the M&RA-approved COSC subject matter and standard terminology in lieu of those provided on the M&RA COSC Web site. The administration of COSC programs should include the following:

- *Training Rosters.* Unit medical personnel create training rosters for all COSC training provided to the unit. These rosters are maintained at the unit's aid station for 3 years.
- *Reporting Requirement for COSC Training.* Unit medical personnel provide training rosters that document individual completion of postdeployment COSC training and require those rosters be provided to their respective S-3s. This information is recorded in the Marine Corps Total Force System Program. The appropriate documentation is also made for Sailors in a page 13 service record entry or as directed by the Chief of Naval Operations.
- *Binnacle Lists, Casualty Reporting, and Patient Tracking.* Personnel diagnosed with a COS-related problem are recorded on the unit binnacle list like any other medical problem. Patients requiring medical evacuation are listed on the unit's casualty/patient tracking report. All entries on these reports

follow unit policy, pertinent Marine Corps instructions, and Health Insurance Portability and Accountability Act regulations.

Unit medical personnel will have the following command and signal responsibilities:

- Medical officers inform their commanders about all unit personnel who exhibit COS symptoms that require evaluation and treatment by an MHP.
- Unit IDC inform their unit leader and unit medical officer about all unit personnel who exhibit COS symptoms that require evaluation and treatment by a medical officer or MHP.
- Field medical technicians inform their unit leader and unit medical officer about all personnel in their companies, platoons, sections, military transition teams, squads, or crews who exhibit COS symptoms that require evaluation and treatment by a medical officer or MHP.

# APPENDIX S

# THE ROLE OF FLEET MEDICAL PERSONNEL IN NAVY OPERATIONAL STRESS CONTROL

The incidence of COS can increase when the operating tempo is high due to multiple "back to back" deployments/extended combat operations. As unit medical personnel, such as general medical officers, flight surgeons, IDC, and hospital corpsmen, provide the primary care for the Sailors and Marines of their unit, they will be the first (in most cases) to evaluate and treat them for COS problems. They are also uniquely positioned to help prevent COS by providing OSC classes to help build resiliency within unit members.

The mission of medical personnel regarding Navy OSC requires that it be prepared to assist in the prevention of COS within the unit and identify and provide initial evaluation and treatment for COS. The mission also requires that medical personnel obtain a mental health professional consultation from or formally refer Service members to a mental health professional when the severity of the COS is beyond the scope of the operational medicine privileges in order to preserve the combat power of the unit.

## Supporting Units and Personnel

Other personnel available to fleet medical personnel may include the carrier psychologist and the mental health department of the local MTF and local Fleet and Family Support Center counselors. Unit chaplains and religious ministry personnel can also provide assistance and COS classes to Marines, Sailors, and their families experiencing COS. Personnel with COS problems beyond the scope of the privileges for the unit medical officer require a mental health professional, such as a carrier psychologist or MTF MHP, consultation or a formal mental health referral.

# Concept of Operations

Since the Navy philosophy emphasizes prevention over treatment and wellness over injury, fleet medical personnel assist the commander by providing the unit with OSC training, identifying those with COS, evaluating and treating with unit-level personnel and assets, and seeking the assistance of an MHP for guidance or formally referring the patient. Unit medical personnel, particularly corpsmen, have served as unit safety representatives and have their "finger on the pulse" of their units. They train together during multiple exercises prior to deployment, deploy together, reside in the same barracks or berthing space, and evaluate/treat all of their other medical conditions in garrison and when underway. Accordingly, unit medical personnel are leaders in the management of COS.

# Fleet Medical Officer Tasks

General medical officers, flight surgeons and IDCs have a responsibility to—

- Attend a Navy-approved OSC training program for health care providers to become proficient with the Navy OSC program as outlined in the NAVADMIN 332/08, *Oversight, Training, and Development of the Operational Stress Control Program*; the stress continuum model; and the stress continuum decision flowchart. Fleet medical providers must be able to use the approved operational stress prevention techniques, provide initial intervention and treatment according to their particular scope of practice, and know when it is appropriate to seek the assistance of or refer the patient to an MHP whether pierside or while deployed.
- Advise commanding officer on the Navy OSC program.
- Inform their commanding officer about all Sailors in the unit who are having significant difficulty managing operational stress using the stress continuum model.
- Update commanding officer on the status of all Sailors from the unit who are being treated by MHPs and provide recommendations on their fitness for duty/deployment.
- Ensure senior medical officers train their unit's junior medical officers, physician assistants, IDC, and corpsmen on their roles and responsibilities in the Navy OSC program and its implementation according to BUMED and Office of the Chief of Naval Operations policy. Implementation information can be found on the Navy Knowledge Online (NKO) OSC

Community of Practice and Naval Center for Combat and Operational Stress Control (NCCOSC) Web sites.

- Work with the unit chaplain to provide/coordinate training for the unit's Sailors, leaders, and families on the OSC topics required by the aforementioned references.
- Understand the local and organic mental health resources, such as the carrier psychologist, deployment health clinic, MTF mental health department, Fleet and Family Support Center, Military OneSource, and NKO OSC Community of Practice and NCCOSC Web sites, that are available to the unit while pierside or deployed and designed to educate the unit, advise the leadership, and ensure timely mental health referrals for their personnel.

# Hospital Corpsmen Tasks

Responsibilities of the hospital corpsmen include—

- Becoming proficient with the Navy OSC program as outlined in the NAVADMIN 332/08, the stress continuum model, and the stress continuum decision flowchart through attending a Navy-approved OSC for healthcare providers training program or training received from their unit medical officer or IDC. Corpsmen must be able to use the approved operational stress prevention techniques, provide initial intervention in accordance with their unit medical officer's guidance, and know when to seek the assistance of their medical officer or MHP.
- Keeping the unit medical officer and division/department leader informed of all Sailors having significant difficulty managing COS using the stress continuum model.
- Ensuring that their unit's junior corpsmen are trained on the Navy OSC program and that they know their roles and responsibilities in its implementation at their unit.
- Providing the training of the Sailors from their unit on the OSC topics required by the aforementioned references and Web sites as directed by their fleet medical officer and unit chaplains and religious ministry personnel.

# Coordinating Instructions

Educational and training materials used to teach the OSC program adhere to NAVADMIN 332/08 and may be found on the NKO

OSC Community of Practice and NCCOSC Web sites. The administration of OSC programs should include the following:

- *Training Rosters.* Fleet medical personnel create training rosters for all OSC training provided to their unit. These rosters are maintained at the unit's aid station for 3 years.
- *Reporting Requirement for OSC Training.* Unit medical personnel provide training rosters that document individual completion of OSC training to their respective education and training departments. This information is documented in a page 13 service record entry or as directed by the Chief of Naval Operations.
- *Binnacle Lists, Casualty Reporting, and Patient Tracking.* Personnel diagnosed with a COS-related problem are recorded on the unit sick call list like any other medical problem. Patients requiring medical evacuation are listed on the unit's casualty/patient tracking report. All entries on these reports follow unit policy, pertinent Office of the Chief of Naval Operations instructions, and Health Insurance Portability and Accountability Act regulations.

Unit medical personnel will have the following command and signal responsibilities:

- Fleet medical officers inform their commanders about all personnel in their unit who exhibit COS symptoms and require evaluation and treatment of an MHP.
- Unit IDC inform their unit leader and unit medical officer about all personnel in their units who exhibit COS symptoms and require evaluation and treatment by a medical officer or MHP.
- Hospital corpsmen inform their unit leader and unit medical officer about all personnel seen in sick call who exhibit COS symptoms and require evaluation and treatment by a medical officer or MHP.

# THE ROLE OF MARINE CORPS FAMILY READINESS OFFICERS

Based on December 2007 demographics data, the active duty Marine Corps includes 179,862 dependants. Married Marines make up 45 percent of the Corps—68.5 percent of officers and 42.5 percent of enlisted—and the average age of a Marine at the birth of his or her first child is 23.5 years. Given the high operating tempo associated with the "long war" and an active duty dependant population that is 96 percent of the active duty Service member population, there is a great need for effective family readiness/wellness and COSC programs.

This appendix is directed at providing commanders, FROs, and other supporting military and civilian staff with guidance on the integration of family readiness/wellness programs with the organization's overall strategy for managing the effects of COS in preparation for, sustainment of, and recovery from combat deployments. Risks associated with failure to thoroughly address family readiness/wellness in the organizational COSC strategy extend beyond the negative impact on unit readiness that results from family disintegration. They bore directly into the personal lives, well-being, and safety of Service members, spouses, children and other relationships.

## Applying Lessons Learned

Marine Corps Order 1754.6A, *Marine Corps Family Team Building*, sets forth the commander's responsibilities with regard to family readiness. Additionally, MCBul 1754, *Primary Duty Family Readiness Officers*, authorizes the establishment of primary duty FROs at battalion level and higher. Traditionally, the collateral duty FRO's scope of authority was limited to the administrative arrangements required of Service members with families prior to deployment, such as family care plans, record of emergency data, wills, or powers of attorney. The Marine Corps Center for Lessons Learned has documented the experience of recurring operational deployments and the effects of COS, which has compelled leaders to call for a more robust approach to family readiness and wellness; hence, primary duty FROs were established and the family readiness and wellness programs enhanced.

There is a direct relationship between the effect of COS in a Service member and the negative impact on that Service member's family and close relations. In cases where the Marine or Sailor is impacted along the continuum to the point of stress injury or illness, a Dirkzwager, Bramsen, Ader and van der Ploeg 2005 study found a high likelihood of psycho-social breakdown within primary interpersonal relationships, ranging from occasional unresolved conflict to chronic substance abuse, complete emotional withdrawal, domestic violence, and homicidal/suicidal behavior.

For the returning warrior, family members provide the main source of psycho-social support. When symptomatic behaviors associated with COS damage primary relationships or when family members hear vivid details of a Service member's traumatic event, family members become vulnerable to stress reaction, injury, or illness. These vicarious stress responses are considered secondary trauma and are particularly devastating to the family unit because the combat veteran is deprived of essential support from the family while they deal with their own reactions. Galovski and Lyons (2004) found that the quality of the relationship and the longevity of the marriage prior to deployment and the spouse's level of dysfunction during the deployment are the best predictors of positive or negative reintegration—even more so than the severity of traumatic stress experienced by the deployed Service member.

# Adapting the Stress Continuum Model and COSC Leadership Functions to Family Readiness Responsibility

Following the concept of secondary trauma, families can be expected to manifest symptoms that reflect the degree of latent dysfunction in the relationship and the stress impact experienced by the returned Marine or Sailor. Family reactions also follow the four zones of the stress continuum model—

- **READY:** Green Zone families may display positive interactions, strong conflict resolution skills, constructive communication, shared household responsibility, confidence in primary relationships, positive interaction with extended network of relationships, and stable school performance for children/work performance for spouse.
- **REACTING:** Yellow Zone families may show occasional protracted conflict or strained communication, diminished contact with extended network of relationships, or occasional disturbance in school/work performance. These reactions diminish over 2 to 3 months.
- **INJURED:** Orange Zone families may experience ongoing conflict that defies resolution, frequent hostility between family members, self-medication, avoidance and emotional withdrawal, cutting ties with extended network of relationships, or fleeing to outside relationships. These reactions do not diminish, but are subtle enough to be concealed from most others.
- **ILL:** Red Zone families may exhibit chronic open conflict, expressed hostility, physical or emotional abuse, separation, self-medication, addiction, divorce, or homicidal/suicidal behavior. These reactions escalate over time.

The establishment of primary duty FROs throughout the Fleet Marine Force can help to lessen or prevent the damaging impact of COS on families. To be most effective, FROs must be involved with families from the outset of predeployment planning through postdeployment reset. They must address not only the administrative requirements of family readiness, but also the need for family wellness training and programs before, during, and after the deployment. The FROs are not family wellness counselors and trainers. Their role is to plan, coordinate, and leverage the considerable resources available through MCCS, MHPs, chaplains, Military OneSource, and other agencies with expertise in the area of family wellness.

Family readiness officers have the following roles with respect to the COSC leadership functions:

- *Strengthen*. Family readiness officers plan and coordinate relationship skills-building opportunities as part of the unit's predeployment and postdeployment reset training. Commanders and senior leaders must expect that married Marines and Sailors and their dependants take part in such training and that single Marines and Sailors have an opportunity for training on this topic as well.
- *Mitigate*. Family readiness officers plan and coordinate for marriage/relationship wellness self-assessments during predeployment and postdeployment reset training to assist families to determine which relationship skills need enhancement. The FROs and unit chaplains refer cases to the appropriate assistance agency or program. Programs include Families OverComing Under Stress, Chaplain's Religious Enrichment Development Operations, MCCS Counseling and Advocacy Program, Marine Corps Family Team Building, mental health, and Military OneSource.
- *Identify*. Family readiness officers plan and coordinate training for dependants to ensure proficiency with the terms, signs, and symptoms associated with COS, stress first aid, and resources available to assist Marines and Sailors dealing with a stress reaction, injury, or illness.
- *Treat*. Family readiness officers, chaplains, and unit medical personnel assist with and refer cases in which families are impacted by COS. They also inform commanders about any degree of domestic violence or abusive or self-destructive behavior.
- *Reintegrate*. Family readiness officers plan and coordinate follow-up and refresher training to insure families remain aware of COS terms, signs, and symptoms and can access assistance resources when needed.

Marines and Sailors undergo mandatory COSC training and, if needed, follow-on care; however, dependants are not required to take part in MOST. As a result, commanders must take every opportunity to invite and motivate family members or significant others to participate in such training and maintain an atmosphere of positive encouragement to seek help when needed.

# APPENDIX U

# THE MARINE OPERATIONAL STRESS TRAINING PROGRAM

The MOST program is based on the stress continuum model and the five core COSC leader functions and covers predeployment, redeployment, and postdeployment. The target audiences are Marine leaders, Marines and Sailors, and family members.

The primary method of delivery is through workshops—whether at the command level or through unit briefings—developed and maintained by HQMC COSC and posted on the M&RA COSC Web site (see fig. U-1). Workshops are updated periodically to reflect new data and trends. Current workshops, sorted by deployment phase, include—

- Predeployment:
  -- Leader Preparation.
  -- Warrior Preparation.
  -- Family Preparation.
- Redeployment:
  -- Leader Transition.
  -- Warrior Transition.
  -- Family Transition.
- Postdeployment:
  -- Leader Transition II.
  -- Warrior Transition II.
  -- Family Transition II.

The Family Preparation and Family Transition briefings are collaborative efforts with Marine Corps Family Team Building. The Warrior Transition II brief is required to be delivered to Marines 60 to 120 days after returning from deployment and is recorded in each Marine's individual record through the Marine Corps Total Force System.

The MOST program identifies those stress injuries and illnesses that would most improve with early intervention and treatment. The most effective way to recognize stress disorders, such as PTSD and anxiety, is by their severe and persistent symptoms. The

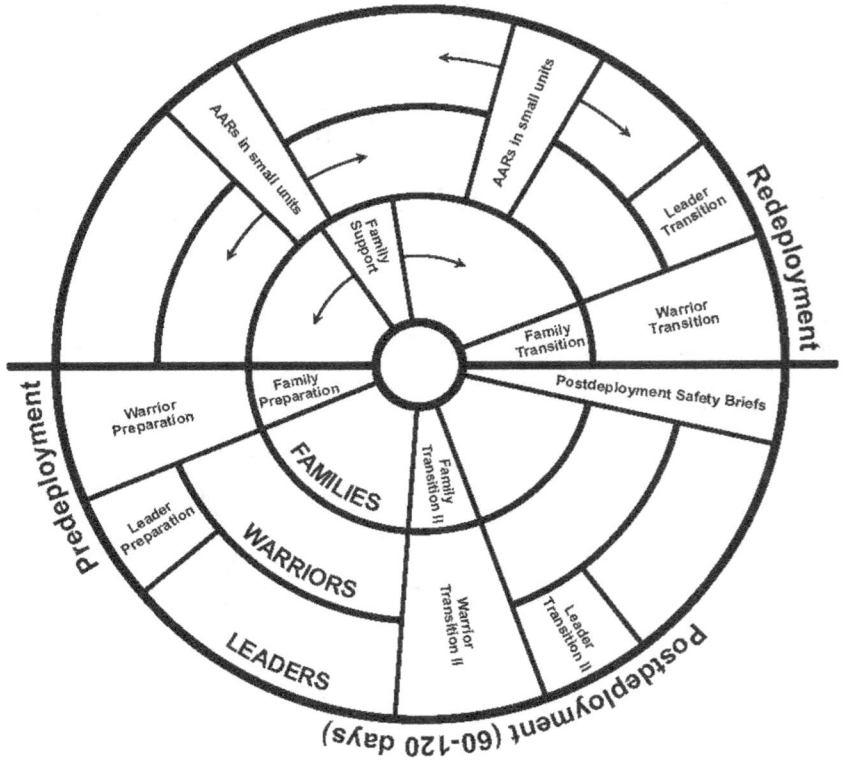

**COSC Awareness Briefs**

- **Predeployment**
  - Leader Preparation
  - Warrior Preparation
  - Family Preparation
- **Before Redeployment**
  - Leader Transition
  - Warrior Transition
  - Family Transition
- **Postdeployment** (60-120 days)
  - Leader Transition II
  - Warrior Transition II
  - Family Transition II

**Figure U-1.** Combat and Operational Stress control Awareness Briefs.

MOST workshops are designed to be interactive, help describe stress problems, and be understood by the target audiences. Each workshop is designed to cover a variety of topics specific for the target audience for a period in the deployment cycle. Goals and objectives of predeployment MOST workshops include—

- Leader Preparation:
  •• Understand stress continuum model.
  •• Understand tactics and timelines of normal coping and resiliency.
  •• Understand five core functions of COSC.
  •• Learn to use stress continuum decision flowchart for stress monitoring.

- •• Know how to prevent and manage stress problems.
- •• Know how to use resources for help when needed.
- • Warrior Preparation:
  - •• Become aware of stress continuum model.
  - •• Understand "stress" and normal coping with stress.
  - •• Recognize and address Yellow, Orange, and Red Zones in self and peers.
  - •• Know where to get help for Orange or Red Zone problems.
- • Family Preparation:
  - •• Understand sources of redeployment and homecoming stress.
  - •• Understand normal process of readapting to home and garrison.
  - •• Become aware of common safety risks postdeployment.
  - •• Know how to reduce risks of postdeployment stress.
  - •• Review stress continuum model.
  - •• Assess self and peers for Orange and Red Zone stress.
  - •• Know where to get help for Orange or Red Zone problems.

Goals and objectives of redeployment MOST workshops include—

- • Leader Transition:
  - •• Understand normal process of readjustment to home and garrison.
  - •• Understand safety risks immediately following deployment.
  - •• Learn ways to reduce risk for postdeployment problems.
  - •• Review stress continuum model.
  - •• Review stress continuum decision flowchart as a tool for postdeployment monitoring.
  - •• Know available resources for help when needed.
- • Warrior Transition:
  - •• Understand sources of redeployment and homecoming stress.
  - •• Understand normal process of readapting to home and garrison.
  - •• Become aware of common safety risks postdeployment.
  - •• Know how to reduce risks of postdeployment stress.
  - •• Review stress continuum model.
  - •• Assess self and peers for Orange and Red Zone stress.
  - •• Know where to get help for Orange or Red Zone problems.
- • Family Transition:
  - •• Understand sources of redeployment and homecoming stress.
  - •• Understand the normal process of readjusting and coping.

- •• Learn tools for coping with family homecoming stress.
- •• Review the stress continuum model as it applies to the entire family.
- •• Assess self and family members for Orange and Red Zone stress.
- •• Learn ways to manage Yellow and Orange Zone stress.
- •• Know where to get help for Yellow, Orange, or Red Zone stress.

Goals and objectives of postdeployment MOST workshops:

- Leader Transition II:
  - •• Review stress continuum model.
  - •• Review five core functions of COSC.
  - •• Review stress continuum decision flowchart for continuous stress monitoring.
  - •• Know the cardinal symptoms of the common postdeployment stress illnesses, such as PTSD, depression, anxiety, or substance abuse.
  - •• Know how to manage Yellow, Orange, and Red Zone stress in units.
  - •• Know how to use resources for help when needed.
- Warrior Transition II:
  - •• Review stress continuum model.
  - •• Review common symptoms of Yellow, Orange, and Red Zone stress.
  - •• Self-assess life functioning and stress level.
  - •• Review techniques for taking care of Yellow and Orange Zone stress in self and peers.
  - •• Know where to get help for Orange or Red Zone problems.
- Family Transition II:
  - •• Review stress continuum model.
  - •• Review common symptoms of Yellow, Orange, and Red Zone stress.
  - •• Self-assess life functioning and stress level.
  - •• Review techniques for taking care of Yellow and Orange Zone stress in self and family members.
  - •• Know where to get help for Orange or Red Zone problems.

All workshops may be delivered by anyone in the unit designated by the commanding officer, but are typically given by a chaplain, medical officer, or staff NCO. The workshops come with speaker's notes and are easy to deliver, but require knowledge of COSC and a thorough understanding of the workshop content prior to leading it.

# APPENDIX V

# NAVY CAREGIVER
# OCCUPATIONAL STRESS CONTROL

The current demands and challenges that military medical personnel face today are dramatically different from those of only a few years ago. Operational and occupational demands are intensified by organizational restructuring, heavier workloads, fewer resources, and sicker patients. Caregivers rarely deploy as a cohesive unit, do not have the protective factors associated with intensive realistic team training, and miss the restorative dwell-time between deployments so critical to combat units. The skills, knowledge, and role expectations that caregivers use in a combat or humanitarian environment are the same ones used in medical centers and clinics, so it is common for caregivers to re-engage in the care of combat casualties when they return to their parent treatment facilities. Consequences of untreated cumulative stress can result in—

- An increased number of medical errors or near misses.
- Physical complaints, such as changes in eating habits, gastrointestinal distress, headache, fatigue, and sleep disorders.
- Change in work habits, such as tardiness/absenteeism.
- Mental and emotional difficulties, such as memory disturbances, anger, self-doubt, isolation, or impaired judgment.
- Accidents.

## The Challenges of Caregiver Stress Control

Evidence suggests that Navy medical personnel are not meeting their own mental health needs or using existing mental health resources before serious consequences occur to themselves or others. The caregiver's code of silence (both moral and professional), dedication to caring for injured Marines and Sailors, and passion to ease suffering increases the need for leaders of caregivers to be vigilant for early stress behaviors.

The dominant stress response paradigm in civilian and Navy literature has several common elements that caregivers need to remember when considering self-care—the sources of job stress, the signs and symptoms of stress, the importance of self-care, and the process of seeking help at the beginning of daily life impairment. Healthcare personnel experience several coping barriers to self-help:

- Prevalent job stress, which produces stress symptoms in all workers so that moderate and high stress look "normal."
- Early stress symptoms, such as fatigue, impaired sleep, and confusion, which decrease self-awareness and ability to engage in self-care.
- Focus on others, for which they receive intrinsic rewards from self-sacrifice and service.
- Stigma, regarding the use of mental health services that are designed for mental illness treatment versus mental health promotion.

Occupational fatigue, compassion fatigue, caregiver stress, and burnout are stress injuries that can result in medical errors, job dissatisfaction, and poor retention. Currently, there is a mix of medical professionals providing some form of compassion fatigue intervention in the major MTFs. Advance practice mental health nurses, clinical social workers, clinical chaplains, and psychiatric technicians currently provide most staff support services. Currently, caregiver interventions are a blend of cognitive behavioral strategies, grief counseling, and stress management strategies that are provided based on the individual skill set of the mental health personnel and the resources available in a command.

# Navy Medicine's Caregiver Occupational Stress Control Program

The Navy Medicine Caregiver OSC program, sometimes called Care for the Caregiver, is one of the Department of Defense resilience initiatives. The Caregiver OSC program works under the three fundamental principles of early recognition, peer intervention, and connection with services as needed and has developed various strategies and resources to assist Navy Medicine caregivers with the operational, occupational, and compassion demands of the job. One of the main strategies for addressing the psychological health needs of caregivers is to develop occupational stress training and intervention strategies for use in a wide range of clinical and operational settings. Core knowledge and skills are needed in the following areas:

- Stress continuum model.
- Occupational stress first aid.
- Buddy care assessment and intervention.
- Self-care/compassion fatigue skills.
- Work environment assessment.
- Education outreach/train the trainer.

# The Five Core OSC Functions for Caregivers

A review of operational lessons learned and AARs highlight the importance of effective leadership in enhancing the mission capabilities of caregivers. Leaders cannot assume that caregivers are not impacted by exposure to operational and garrison duties. Leaders who are responsible for caregivers need to consider the following adaptations of the five core COSC leadership functions to maintain caregiver mission readiness:

- *Strengthen.* Caregiver training typically focuses on the "just in time" elements of the mission or the clinical environment. The warrior-healer duality of the caregiver role needs to be acknowledged and practiced in the training. Training evolutions need to include AARs that incorporate the usual who, what, where, and how of the exercise and a discussion of the meaning of that event to the caregiver role or expectations. Building cohesion is paramount because caregivers rarely participate in the full cycle of predeployment training and may need leader support to be welcomed into an established cohesive unit.
- *Mitigate.* Caregivers are often considered "containers of resources" in the leaky bucket stress metaphor. As a "resource," there is a risk that they may not be meeting their own physical, social, mental, and spiritual needs. Leaders should remember to include caregivers in the practices to conserve physical health and well-being and consider having caregivers from other units engage each other in a process of mutual assessment and support.
- *Identify.* Caregivers are very adept at avoiding or minimizing responses to screening questionnaires and other early warning assessment tools. Leaders must apply stress first aid actions to address their concerns and trust their own assessments.

- *Treat.* The stress first aid strategies are as effective for caregivers as they are for other Sailors and Marines, except that caregivers are usually engaged in their roles and may not show symptoms of stress injury until after the last patient is treated or they have turned over their responsibilities to the next shift. Leaders must observe caregivers during periods of quiet and solitude following intense activity or during prolonged and fatiguing care experiences. Being connected and competent are critical intervening qualities used to support caregivers.
- *Reintegrate.* Postdeployment reintegration is particularly challenging for caregivers. They deploy as individual augmentees from their parent commands, become part of a cohesive unit, must leave it and return to their parent command, and become part of a new unit. Since caregivers have their own stressors and may place more emphasis on getting "back to work," they may ignore affecting a purposeful reintegration. Operational deployment experiences change a caregiver's tolerance for an "unimportant issue," such as administrative processes or rules that do not appear to improve patient care. Leaders may consider phasing in work schedules and delaying collateral duty assignments as part of a caregiver's postdeployment or poststress injury reintegration.

# GLOSSARY

## Section I. Abbreviations and Acronyms

AAR. . . . . . . . . . . . . . . . . . . . . . . . . . . . . . . . . . . . . . . . . . . . . . . . . after action review
BUMED. . . . . . . . . . . . . . . . . . . . . . . . . . . . . . . . . .Bureau of Medicine and Surgery
COS. . . . . . . . . . . . . . . . . . . . . . . . . . . . . . . . . . . . . . . combat and operational stress
COSC. . . . . . . . . . . . . . . . . . . . . . . . . . . . . . . combat and operational stress control
FRO. . . . . . . . . . . . . . . . . . . . . . . . . . . . . . . . . . . . . . . . . .family readiness officer
GCS. . . . . . . . . . . . . . . . . . . . . . . . . . . . . . . . . . . . . . . . . . .Glasgow Coma Scale
HQMC. . . . . . . . . . . . . . . . . . . . . . . . . . . . . . . . . . . . Headquarters, Marine Corps
IDC . . . . . . . . . . . . . . . . . . . . . . . . . . . . . . . . . . . . .independent duty corpsmen
IED . . . . . . . . . . . . . . . . . . . . . . . . . . . . . . . . . . . improvised explosive device
KSA. . . . . . . . . . . . . . . . . . . . . . . . . . . . . . . . . . . knowledge, skill, and attitude
M&RA. . . . . . . . . . . . . . . . . . . . . . . . . . . . .Manpower and Reserve Affairs (HQMC)
MACE . . . . . . . . . . . . . . . . . . . . . . . . . . . . . Military Acute Concussion Evaluation
MCBul. . . . . . . . . . . . . . . . . . . . . . . . . . . . . . . . . . . . . . Marine Corps bulletin
MCCS . . . . . . . . . . . . . . . . . . . . . . . . . . . . . Marine Corps Community Services
MEF. . . . . . . . . . . . . . . . . . . . . . . . . . . . . . . . . . . . . Marine expeditionary force
MHP . . . . . . . . . . . . . . . . . . . . . . . . . . . . . . . . . . . . . . . .mental health provider
MOST . . . . . . . . . . . . . . . . . . . . . . . . . . . . . . Marine Operational Stress Training
mTBI. . . . . . . . . . . . . . . . . . . . . . . . . . . . . . . . . . . . mild traumatic brain injury
MTF. . . . . . . . . . . . . . . . . . . . . . . . . . . . . . . . . . . . . . . military treatment facility
NAVADMIN. . . . . . . . . . . . . . . . . . . . . . . . . . . . . . . . naval administrative message
NCO. . . . . . . . . . . . . . . . . . . . . . . . . . . . . . . . . . . . . . noncommissioned officer
NCCOSC. . . . . . . . . . . . . . . Naval Center for Combat and Operational Stress Control
NEC. . . . . . . . . . . . . . . . . . . . . . . . . . . . . . . . . . . . . .Navy enlisted classification
NKO . . . . . . . . . . . . . . . . . . . . . . . . . . . . . . . . . . . .Navy Knowledge Online
OSC. . . . . . . . . . . . . . . . . . . . . . . . . . . . . . . . . . . . .operational stress control
OSCAR . . . . . . . . . . . . . . . . . . . . . . . . Operational Stress Control and Readiness
PFA . . . . . . . . . . . . . . . . . . . . . . . . . . . . . . . . . . . . . . psychological first aid
PTSD. . . . . . . . . . . . . . . . . . . . . . . . . . . . . . . . . . . posttraumatic stress disorder
RMT . . . . . . . . . . . . . . . . . . . . . . . . . . . . . . . . . . . . religious ministry team
S-3 . . . . . . . . . . . . . . . . . . . . . . . . battalion or regiment operations section
SPRINT. . . . . . . . . . . . . . . . . . . . . . . . . .special psychiatric rapid intervention team
TBI. . . . . . . . . . . . . . . . . . . . . . . . . . . . . . . . . . . . . . . . . traumatic brain injury
THR. . . . . . . . . . . . . . . . . . . . . . . . . . . . . . . . . . . . . . . . . . . target heart rate

## Section II. Terms and Definitions

**adaptive coping**—The normal, temporary process of coping with a stressor, usually by either changing oneself physically and mentally to be better suited for that particular stressor or by becoming numb to the mental and physical effects of that stressor. Stress adaptive coping is always temporary and it always fades after the stressor is no longer experienced.

**after action review**—A traditional method for leaders to gather and share information in a unit, after any operational or training event, about what went right, what didn't go right, and why events proceeded as they did. After action reviews disseminate lessons learned in order to improve performance. Also called **AAR**. (Proposed for inclusion in the next edition of MCRP 5-12C.)

**combat and operational stress**—The expected and predictable emotional, intellectual, physical, and/or behavioral reactions of Service members who have been exposed to stressful events in combat or noncombat military operations. Combat stress reactions vary in quality and severity as a function of operational conditions, such as intensity, duration, rules of engagement, leadership, effective communication, unit morale, unit cohesion, and perceived importance of the mission. Also called **COS**. (Proposed for inclusion in the next edition of MCRP 5-12C.)

**combat and operational stress control**—Leader actions and responsibilities to promote resilience and psychological health in military units and individuals, including families, exposed to the stress of combat or other military operations. Also called **COSC**.

**combat and operational stress first aid**—A set of tools with three simple aims: **(1)** preserve life, **(2)** prevent further harm, and **(3)** promote recovery. Combat and operational stress first aid components include the "seven Cs": check, coordinate, cover, calm, connect, competence, and confidence.

**combat stress**—Changes in physical or mental functioning or behavior resulting from the experience or lethal force or its aftermath. These changes can be positive and adaptive or they can be negative, including distress or loss of normal functioning.

**family readiness officer**—A staff officer assigned to commands down to the level of battalion or equivalent who is responsible to address the administrative requirements of family readiness and the need for family wellness training and programs before, during, and after deployment. Also called **FRO**.

**first aid**—A set of procedures for the initial premedical care of injuries and illnesses.

**fortitude**—The ability to encounter danger or bear pain or adversity without faltering.

**improvised explosive device**—A device placed or fabricated in an improvised manner incorporating destructive, lethal, noxious, pyrotechnic, or incendiary chemicals and designed to destroy, incapacitate, harass, or distract. It may incorporate military stores, but is normally devised from nonmilitary components. Also called **IED**. (JP 1-02)

**knowledge, skill, and attitude**—A training term that describes the necessary component goals of a particular training activity. Also called **KSA**.

**Marine Operational Stress Training**—The Marine Corps' program for deployment cycle-specific combat and operational stress training for leaders, Marines, and families. The primary method of delivery is command-level and unit briefings and workshops designed to help prevent, identify, and effectively manage combat operational stress problems at all levels. Also called **MOST**.

**mental health**—The absence of significant distress or impairment due to mental illness. Mental health is a prerequisite for psychological health. Also called **MH**.

**mental health provider**—Licensed independent providers credentialed and authorized (privileged) to provide formal mental health services without supervision. Typically, professions filling this role include psychiatrists, psychologists, licensed clinical social workers, and mental health clinical nurse practitioners. Also called **MHP**.

**military treatment facility**—A facility established for the purpose of furnishing medical and/or dental care to eligible individuals. Also called **MTF**. (JP 1-02)

**mission-oriented protective posture**—A flexible system of protection against chemical, biological, radiological, and nuclear contamination. This posture requires personnel to wear only that protective clothing and equipment (mission-oriented protective posture gear) appropriate to the threat level, work rate imposed by the mission, temperature, and humidity. Also called **MOPP**. (JP 1-02)

**noncommissioned officer**—A small unit leader in the Marine Corps, usually an E-4 or E-5. Also called **NCO**.

**operational stress**—Changes in physical or mental functioning or behavior resulting from the experience or consequences of military operations other than combat, during peacetime or war, and on land, at sea, or in the air.

**operational (or occupational) stress control**—Leader actions and responsibilities to promote resilience and psychological health in military units and individuals, including family members, exposed to the stress of routine or wartime military operations in noncombat environments. Also called **OSC**.

**Operational Stress Control and Readiness**—A Marine Corps program that assigns mental health personnel directly as organic assets in ground combat units at the level of regiments, rather than attaching them to external medical treatment facilities or combat stress teams. Also called **OSCAR**.

**operational stress injuries**—Persistent changes in the brain and mind caused by combat or operational stress that exceeds in intensity or duration, the ability of the individual to adapt.

**petty officer**—A noncommissioned officer in the Navy. Also called **PO**.

**postdeployment health reassessment**—A self-report screening tool used to identify Service members experiencing medical or combat stress problems or injuries 3 to 6 months postdeployment.

**posttraumatic stress disorder**—An anxiety disorder resulting from exposure to extreme trauma. Also called **PTSD**.

**psychological first aid**—Psychological support and assistance provided in the immediate aftermath of a traumatic event. Also called **PFA**.

**psychological health**—Wellness in mind, body, and spirit. Also called **PH**.

**religious ministry team**—A team that consists of the chaplain(s) religious program specialist(s), and other designated command members (e.g., chaplain's assistants, civilian staff, appointed lay leaders). Each religious ministry team's (RMT's) composition will be determined by the command's mission and table of organization. Each RMT will have a minimum of one assigned Navy chaplain. Also called **RMT**. (MCRP 5-12C)

**religious program specialist**—A Navy enlisted assistant who supports a chaplain in planning, programming, administering, and coordinating the command religious program. A religious program specialist is a combatant who provides force protection and physical security for a chaplain in operational environments. (This term and its definition are proposed for inclusion in the next edition of MCRP 5-12C by MCWP 6-12.)

**resilience**—The process of preparing for, recovering from, and adjusting to life in the face of stress, adversity, trauma, or tragedy.

**seven Cs of combat and operational stress first aid**—A memory aid (check, coordinate, cover, calm, connect, competence, and confidence).

**special psychiatric rapid intervention team**—A multidisciplinary Navy team that provides intervention in maritime mishaps, stability and contingency operations, terrorist attacks, and natural disasters. The teams consist of two psychiatrists, two clinical psychologists, one chaplain, one psychiatric nurse, and four hospital corpsmen psychiatric technicians. Also called **SPRINT**.

**stress illness**—A diagnosable mental disorder resulting from an unhealed stress injury that worsens over time to cause significant disability in one or more spheres of life.

**stress injury**—More severe and persistent distress or loss of functioning caused by disruptions to the integrity of the brain, mind, or spirit after exposure to overwhelming stressors. Stress injuries are invisible but literal wounds caused by stress, but like more visible physical wounds, they usually heal, especially if given proper care.

**stressor**—Any mental or physical challenge or set of challenges.

**stress reaction**—The common, temporary, and often necessary experience of mild distress or changes in functioning due to stress from any cause.

**traumatic brain injury**—A brain injury caused by a blow or jolt to the head or a penetrating head injury that disrupts the normal function of the brain. Also called **TBI**. (Centers for Disease Control and Prevention)

**willpower**—The motivation to convert mental strength into courageous behavior.

# REFERENCES AND RELATED PUBLICATIONS

## Geneva Conventions of 1949

Convention (I) for the Amelioration of the Condition of the Wounded and Sick in Armed Forces in the Field, 12 August 1949.

## Chief of Naval Operations Instructions (OPNAVINSTs)

| | |
|---|---|
| 1300.14_ | Suitability Screening for Overseas and Remote Duty Assignment |
| 3591.1_ | Small Arms Training and Qualification |

## Department of Defense Instructions (DODIs)

| | |
|---|---|
| 1332.38 | Discharge Review Board (DRB) Procedures and Standards |
| 5200.2_ | Personnel Security Program |
| 6130.4 | Medical Standards for Appointment, Enlistment, or Induction in the Armed Forces |
| 6490.1 | Mental Health Evaluations of Members of the Armed Forces |
| 6490.4 | Requirements for Mental Health Evaluations of Members of the Armed Forces |

## Marine Corps Bulletins (MCBuls)

| | |
|---|---|
| 1754 | Primary Duty Family Readiness Officers |
| 6490 | Combat Operational Stress Control (COSC) Program |

## Marine Corps Orders (MCOs)

| | |
|---|---|
| 1754.6A | Marine Corps Family Team Building |
| P1300.8_ | Marine Corps Personnel Assignment Policy |

## Memoranda and Correspondence

Assistant Secretary of Defense for Health Affairs Memorandum of 7 Nov 06, *Policy Guidance for Deployment-Limiting Psychiatric Conditions and Medications.*

Chief of Naval Operations Memorandum of 01 May 08, *Immediate Policy Implementation—Mental Health Question, Standard Form (SF) 86, Questionnaire for National Security Positions.*

Commanding Generals I MEF, II MEF, III MEF Joint letter, Tri-MEF Combat Operational Stress Conference

Headquarters, Multi-National Corps-Iraq, Baghdad, Iraq. *Multi-National Corps-Iraq (MNC-I) Policy on Mild Traumatic Brain Injury.*

Secretary of Defense Memorandum of 18 Apr 08, *Policy Implementation—Mental Health Question, Standard Form (SF) 86, Questionnaire for National Security Positions.*

## Navy Administrative Message (NAVADMIN)

| | |
|---|---|
| 332/08 | Oversight, Training, and Development of the Operational Stress Control Program |

## Navy Bureau of Medicine and Surgery Instructions (BUMEDINSTs)

| | |
|---|---|
| 3301.3_ | Medical Operations Center (MOC) |
| 6440.6 | Mobile Medical Augmentation Readiness Team (MMART) Manual |

## Secretary of the Navy Instructions (SECNAVINSTs)

| | |
|---|---|
| 1850.4_ | Department of the Navy (DON) Disability Evaluation Manual |
| 1910.4_ | Enlisted Administrative Separations |
| 1920.6_ | Administrative Separations of Officers |
| 5510.30_ | Department of the Navy Personnel Security Program |
| 6320.24_ | Mental Health Evaluations of Members of the Armed Forces |

## Books and Articles Cited

Corrigan, Patrick. How Stigma Interferes with Mental Health Care. *American Psychologist*. 2004; 59(7): 614–625.

Cushman, R. E. Battle Replacements. *Marine Corps Gazette*, November 1947: 46–47.

Dirkzwager, A. J. E., I. Bramsen, H. Ader, and H. M. van der Pleog. Secondary Traumatization in Partners and Parents of Dutch Peacekeeping Soldiers. *Journal of Family Psychology*. 2005; 19, 217–226.

Drescher, Kent D., Smith, Mark W., and Foy, David. Spirituality and Readjustment Following War-Zone Experiences. In C. R. Figley, and W. P. Nash, (Eds.). *Combat Stress Injury: Theory, Research, and Management*. New York: Routledge, 2007.

Galovski, Tara and Judith A Lyons. Psychological Sequelae of Combat Violence: A Review of the Impact of PTSD on the Veteran's Family and Possible Interventions. *Journal of Aggression and Violent Behavior*. 2004; 9, 477–501.

Grossman, Dave. *On Killing*. New York: Back Bay Books; Little, Brown & Company, 1995.

Jones, Frank D. Psychiatric Lessons of War. In: Jones, F.D., Sparacino, L.R., Wilcox, V.L., Rothberg, J.M., Stokes, J.W., eds. *War Psychiatry*. Washington, DC: Borden Institute; 1995

Hilton, S.M., Service, D.B., Stander, V.A., Werbel, A.D., Chavez, B.R. Department of the Navy Suicide Incident Report (DONSIR): *Summary of 1999–2007 Findings*. Naval Research Center, 2009.

Hobfoll, Stevan E. *Stress, Culture, and Community: The Psychology and Philosophy of Stress*. New York: Plenum Press, 1998.

Keinan, Maj R., Keren, LTC Tzur. The Construction of the "Common Truth"—Socio-Psychological Aspects of Combat After Action Review. Presentation at the September 2007 Military Psychology Center Conference, Tel Aviv, Israel.

Lerner, Paul. *Hysterical Men: War, Psychiatry, and the Politics of Trauma in Germany, 1890–1930*, Ithaca: Cornell University Press, 2003.

Marshall, S. L. A. *Men Against Fire: The Problem of Battle Command*. Norman, OK: University of Oklahoma Press, 1947.

Maslow, Abraham. A Theory of Human Motivation. *Psychological Review*, volume 50. 1943; 370–396.

Mattis, LtGen James N., Stalder, LtGen Keith J., Zilmer, LtGen Richard C. Tri-MEF Working Group. 12 September 2007.

Moran, Lord C. M. W. *Anatomy of Courage*. Boston: Houghton Mifflin Company, 1967 (originally published 1945).

Morgan, Charles A., Wang, S., Mason, J., Southwick, Steven M., Fox, P., Hazlett, G., Charney, Dennis S., and Greenfield, G. Hormone Profiles in Humans Experiencing Military Survival Training. *Biological Psychiatry*. 47, 2000; 891–901.

Nash, William P., Steenkamp, Maria, Conoscenti, Laura, and Litz, Brett. The Stress Continuum Model: A Military Organizational Approach to Resilience and Recovery. Steven Southwick, Dennis Charney, Matthew Friedman, and Brett Litz (Eds.), *Resilience: Responding to Challenges Across the Lifespan*. New York: Cambridge University Press, in press.

Pfaff, Donald W., Martin, Eugene M., Ribeiro, Ana C. Relations between Mechanisms of CNS Arousal and Mechanisms of Stress. *Stress*. The Rockefeller University: New York, 2007.

Preamble to the Constitution of the World Health Organization as adopted by the International Health Conference, New York, 19–22 June, 1946; signed on 22 July 1946 by the representatives of 61 States (Official Records of the World Health Organization, no. 2, p. 100) and entered into force on 7 April 1948.

Shay, Jonathan. *Odysseus in America: Combat Trauma and the Trials of Homecoming*. New York: Scribner, 2002.

Shephard, Ben. *War of Nerves: Soldiers and Psychiatrists in the Twentieth Century*. Cambridge, Mass: Harvard University Press, 2001

Van Dongen, Hans P. A., Maislin, Greg, Mullington, J. M., and Dinges, D. F. The Cumulative Cost of Additional Wakefulness: Dose-Response Effects on Neurobehavioral Functions and Sleep Physiology from Chronic Sleep Restriction and Total Sleep Deprivation. *Sleep*. 2, 2003; 117–126.

## Additional Resources and Related Publications

Department of Defense Directive 6490.5, *Combat Stress Control (CSC) Programs*

Department of Defense Inspector General Report 96–079, *Evaluation Report on the Management of Combat Stress Control in the Department of Defense*.

Department of Veterans Affairs, Department of Defense, VA/DOD *Clinical Practice Guidelines for the Management of Post-Traumatic Stress*, January 2004. Available at http://www.oqp.med.va.gov/cpg/ptsd/ptsd_Base.htm.

Fals-Stewart, William. When Family Members Go to War—Systematic Perspective on Harm and Healing. *Journal of Family Psychology*. 19, 2005; 233–236.

Figley, Charles R. and Nash, William P. *Combat Stress Injury: Theory, Research, and Management*. Routledge: New York, 2007.

Knox, James and Price, David H. *The Changing American Military Family: Opportunities for Social Work*. Social Service Review. 69, 1995; 479–497.

Kraft, Heidi S. *Rule Number 2: Lessons I learned in a Combat Hospital*. Little, Brown, and Company: New York, 2007.

Litz, Brett T. *Early Intervention for Trauma and Traumatic Loss*. Guilford Press: New York, 2004.

Marine Corps Community Services. Marine Corps Community Services Demographics Update, December 2007: *The Marine Corps "A Young and Vigorous Force."* http://www.usmc-mccs.org/aboutmccs/downloads/pom/Demographicsupdate.pdf.

Nash, William P. U.S. Marine Corps and Navy Combat and Operational Stress Continuum Model: A Tool for Leaders. In E.C. Ritchie (Ed.), *Combat and Operational Behavioral Health*. Textbooks of Military Medicine series. Washington DC: Borden Institute (in press).

Schmidt, Donald E., Keating, John P. Human Crowding and Personal Control: An Integration of the Research. *Psychological Bulletin*. 86, 1979; 680–700.

Shay, Jonathan. Ethical Standing for Commander Self-Care: The Need for Sleep. *Parameters*, Summer 1998; 93–105.

Shay, Jonathan. *Trust: Lubricant for "Friction" in Military Operations*. November 1998.

Stamm, B. Hudnall, *Secondary Traumatic Stress: Self-Care Issues for Clinicians, Researchers, and Educators*. Sidran Press: Lutherville, MD, 1999.

Tubesing, Nancy L. and Tubesing, Donald A. *Structures Exercises in Stress Management*, Volumes 1–5, and Structured Exercises in Wellness Promotion, Volumes 1–5. Whole Person Associates: Duluth, MN, 1994.

United States Department of Veterans Affairs. National Center for Posttraumatic Stress Disorder. http://www.ncptsd.va.gov/ncmain/.